GOD'S ANSWER TO FAT
...LOØSE IT!

by Frances Hunter

published by
Hunter Ministries
1600 Townhurst
Houston, Texas 77043

1st Printing December, 1975 25,000
2nd Printing January, 1976 25,000
3rd Printing March, 1976 50,000
4th Printing May, 1976 100,000
5th Printing July, 1976 100,000
6th Printing October, 1976 100,000
7th Printing April, 1977 100,000
8th Printing November, 1977 100,000

ISBN 0-917726-00-6
Scripture quotations are taken from:

The Authorized King James Version (KJV)
The Living Bible, Paraphrased. Tyndale House Publishers, Wheaton, Illinois, 1971. All references not specified are from the Living Bible.
Revised Standard Version of the Bible, Zondervan Publishing House, Inc., Grand Rapids, Michigan.

Dedicated to my daughter Joan in whom I created a "fat" problem, but who loves me in spite of my faults.

FOREWORD

People who write forewords glow from ear to ear, and usually are not believed! It's a literary "love-in," or between Frances and I, it's a fanatic's fan club.

I've read this book line by line, word by word. It's alive and well, and if YOU are overweight, it loves YOU.

It's also riddled with technical inaccuracies and awash with personal conjectures and suppositions, but it's beautiful, and it's honest and its author is alive and well and substantially thinner.

Before I became a Christian, I was weight watcher's Public Enemy No. 1 International! I sold the idea of excess and became successful at it. To eat rich was "in," but to look fat was "out." That's Satan's way of substituting failure and guilt for your God given joy and peace.

FRANCES HAS WON, SHE IS THE VICTOR!!! We experts can have all our wisdom of the world and snicker behind sticky fingers, but the fact is Frances did it and has recorded how she did it!

All you have to do is read, see your own overlarded life, and be convicted by her insight and experience to give your appetite to God. After all, he's a pretty good nutritionalist for the creator of our universe and he has an excellent reason for delivering the goods . . . . . HE LOVES YOU!

Graham Kerr

P.S. One of the inaccuracies is in the word "probably" on page 43, line 2.

SPECIAL INSTRUCTIONS:

Before you start to read this book, would you get a pencil or a felt tip pen?

I want you to underline all the parts that particularly apply to you and put a star or a check mark at the top of the page.

When you have finished reading the book, would you go back and reread those parts? I think you'll discover it will do something for you.

Pull that sweet tooth out in the name of Jesus! Put a wisdom tooth in its place.

Frances

Frances

TABLE OF CONTENTS

THE GREAT CHRISTIAN FIB 9
THE GREAT AWAKENING 15
HOW DID IT START AND WHERE DOES IT END? ... 27
WISDOM AND KNOWLEDGE COME GALLOPING IN 43
GLUTTONY 59
WHERE DO WE GO FROM HERE? 65
THE DEVIL IS A "SWEET" LIAR 67
THE GREAT SUBSTITUTION 75
LEARN THE LAW! 85
WHY DON'T I "WANT" TO LOSE WEIGHT? 93
THE WRAP UP 101
NUTRITIVE VALUE OF FOODS (USDA Bulletin No. 72) 107
SKINNY MINNIE RECIPES 143

CHAPTER I

THE GREAT CHRISTIAN FIB

I've been on every kind of diet there is! I've been on the water diet, I've been on the grapefruit diet, I've been on a banana diet, I've been on a liquid diet, I've been on a solid diet, I've been on a fruit salad diet, I've been on an egg diet, I've been on a high protein diet, I've been on a low protein diet, I've been on a no carbohydrate diet, I've been on an ALL carbohydrate diet!

I have tried all kinds of exercising machines. I have gone to spas and had myself absolutely pummeled and beaten to death! I have ridden on stationary bicycles until I was so sore and tired that I could hardly get home. I have been literally shaken to pieces by electric belts. I have laid on machines which roll and bump and thump and make you black and blue. I have baked in saunas, wet and dry, until I was so weak I had to eat a hot fudge sundae to get enough strength to get home. I have stood in scalding whirlpool baths until I nearly had heat exhaustion. I have done everything any person could possibly do to try to stop this up-down-up-down-up-down (mostly up) weight. Before I became a Christian I took every kind of pill in the world you could think about, trying to lose weight. None of them ever seemed to be very effective. Nothing ever worked!

I had been on one of these diets and had lost a considerable amount of weight before I met Charles, and then we were gloriously married and gloriously happy! I began, for the first time in my life, to have leisure time. For the first time in my life I didn't have to make a living for myself and my children, and I had a husband to take care of and protect me. I just loved it! Like many brides, I began the "cooking thing." Charles has never had a problem with weight because he has never had a tremendous desire for food. He would say to me, "Honey, I wish you wouldn't cook such big meals. We don't need this much to eat." And I'd say, "Oh, honey, I love you and I want to spoil you and that's why I want to give you some real good meals." Charles gained a little bit of weight, but I gained a lot!

Being a Christian, I decided that God loved me just as I was, and anyway, when you got to be over 50 you just naturally gained weight!

Charles and I continued to share around the country and unfortunately as an evangelist you have the most difficult time in the world establishing any kind of eating habits because food is mostly eaten late at night. We would eat one meal in the afternoon and then, after a miracle service, I would be starving because I had one meal during the day and so, we would look for some place open late at night. If we even managed to find a place open, it was where you could get hamburgers and french fries — the two things that are probably the worst in the world for anybody who's trying to keep their figure. Many times we couldn't even find a hamburger place open so we would raid the candy machine at the motel where we were staying — sometimes eating 2, 3 and 4 candy bars. It may sound like 4 candy bars is a lot for supper; but it isn't, because it doesn't satisfy you in the least, and it certainly can put weight on you. Little by little I continued to gain weight.

I don't know if it was during this period that Charles ate less than I did or if he just has a metabolism that burns up food faster than I do. He did not have the weight problem that I had, although he did gain about 8 pounds the first five years of our marriage. I GAINED A DISGUSTING TOTAL OF 50!!!

I refused to accept the fact that my dress sizes were getting larger and larger all the time. I got to the point where it was almost impossible to buy a dress just because there were so few in the size I had to wear. The ones I owned had all been "shrunk" by the cleaners! I continued to console myself by saying, "Well, you really do get fatter when you're old, but God loves me just exactly the way I am, and Charles loves me, and that's the only thing that's important." But inside me there was a gnawing that wouldn't stop. It really grew when I got a glimpse of myself in a store window and I sometimes wondered where it would all end.

Do you want me to share something funny with you? We all do silly little things. I used to say "I don't know why I gain weight." Did you ever say that? Then I'd go on, "Charles eats a lot more than I do and yet he never has a weight problem and I do. I must have a glandular problem." Sound familiar? "I don't know why I gain weight. I eat like a bird." But what kind of bird?. . . A 500 pound canary? That's exactly the way I ate. Just exactly like a bird — but oh, what a BIG bird he was!

Charles began to suggest that it might help if I would cut down on eating, but isn't it peculiar when our loved one mentions this, it has a devilish effect on us? Did you know that? Because then we start the Great Christian Fib. I'd say to Charles "I don't understand why I'm gaining so much." We would sit down to eat dinner and we'd both have a steak and a salad. What's wrong with that? Nothing, except . . . the steak was always cooked in butter and when I put it on the plate I put more on the top to melt so it would be real juicy and good. We always had a huge salad because I didn't want to eat anything fattening like potatoes. Great, except . . . I just loaded it with oil and lots of times tiny little hunks of cheese, croutons, bacon bits, etc.

I have always heard that steak and salad were the two most excellent foods to eat while dieting, so we had steak and salad two times a day, and I got fatter and fatter! No one ever told me to eat only 3½ ounces of steak per meal, so at each meal we would have an 8 to 12 ounce steak. NO WONDER I CONTINUED TO GAIN! Many times during the daytime Charles would be so busy at his CPA practice that he didn't have time to eat lunch, but I always saw to it that I took time out to eat a real good reducer's lunch: a great big salad, gobbed with oil, and a nice juicy steak with butter. I continued to gain, and GAIN AND GAIN!!!

About this time I began to wonder if I had a tumor in my stomach. It seemed that all my weight congregated right in the front and my stomach looked about the size of a basketball! One day I said to Charles, "Honey, do you think I could possibly have a tumor in my stomach? I don't have very much weight around the hip area, but my stomach really is something." It can be very embarrassing when you're getting close to 60 to have someone walk up to you and ask if you're expecting a baby. *It happened to me!* (Just call me Sarah) I wondered if I really ought to go to a doctor and check it out. Charles said, "Well, let's just pray and ask God to take care of this and we'll believe that there's nothing wrong with you." I went and bought a tighter girdle!

I began to puff when we went upstairs. I noticed that when we went into a church if we had more than three steps to walk up I'd be puffing by the time we got there. When we walked up onto the rostrum I was puffing and Charles would have to start the talking until I got my breath. I just attributed this to the fact that I was getting older. Little did I realize that I was letting fat congregate around my heart and it was literally squeezing my life out. Every once in a while Charles would say to me, "Honey, don't you think you could really cut down on your food just a little bit, because I think you'd feel so much better if you did." Then Charles began to say a little more about my weight. He said, "Honey, I really think it would be so much better for you if you would try to cut down — even just a little bit." So I started cutting down. And Charles couldn't understand why I didn't lose weight because I didn't eat nearly as much as he did. And I'd say, "Well, honey, you eat so much more than I do, why don't you gain weight like I do?" But you know what? The foodaholic doesn't like anyone talking about his eating habits any more than the alcoholic likes anyone talking about his drinking habits. That's why the foodaholic and the alcoholic begin to eat and drink in secret. We don't want anyone talking about our habits! And that's what I did!

I began to eat in secret! I didn't tell Charles that before he came home I would eat half a pound of cheddar cheese! Together with two bags of corn chips! I would get so hungry when I was making dessert for him that I would make three extra ones and eat them before he got home. I knew how upset he would be if he saw me eating four desserts so I only ate one with him. Before he came home I nibbled and snacked on corn chips, potato chips, cheese dip, cookies, candy, and all kinds of little goodies, so no wonder by the time he got there I didn't eat nearly as much as he did. I was still perfectly capable of enjoying a complete meal even after eating all of this. I'll never be able to understand it except I want to tell you that I am a "foodaholic" and I have always been and I will always be, but with God's help, this foodaholic is going to let Jesus control her appetite from now on!

I wonder why it is so many of us think that just because we eat in secret we're not going to gain weight. Why is it we think when we furtively sneak something in the kitchen before our husband gets home, it doesn't count? Why is it we can eat a sweet roll in the car on the way home from the bakery and think it's calorieless? Why is it we always think we'll diet "tomorrow" and just because we're going to do that, what we eat today won't show up on the scale? It's the funniest thing — you can stand in a kitchen alone and eat the most fattening thing in the world and think it won't count so far as weight is concerned, just because no one is watching! Have you ever done that? I did that so many times and when I look back at it now I think it's absolutely hysterical!!!

CHAPTER II
THE GREAT AWAKENING!

I began to see pictures of me and I didn't like the way they looked! Even when I looked at myself in the mirror I thought "That doesn't look like my face. I wonder what's the matter with me." And the more frustrated I got, the more weight I gained. Then I decided that possibly I was retaining water in my old age and my face was just puffing up because of the excess fluid that I was carrying. Isn't it amazing how we'll never admit the truth? Isn't it amazing that we'll never admit that we just plain eat too much and that we are foodaholics? I say it now and I will continue to say it . . . "I am a foodaholic, but I will from this day on let Jesus, instead of my own flesh, have control of my appetite."

People often take pictures of us when we're on tours. Many of them are kind enough (or unkind enough) to send them to us. I've looked at pictures and thought "I don't believe it," and then I'd say "I've got to do something about this." I would decide that I was going to diet and then you know what would happen? By noontime I was so hungry that I was willing to eat anything I could find . . . and I did! I ate anything and everything that came in sight!

I would see pictures in magazines after Charles and I

had been to a regional convention, and I shuddered when I saw most of them, but there was one crowning one that really threw me for a loop. We went to the Christian Retreat in Bradenton, Florida, and the photographer took a picture of us. It was a side view which showed my big fat stomach at its very largest! I took a second look and thought "I don't believe it. I cannot believe this is the way I look," and for the first time I started to get honest about my weight.

Then ANOTHER very interesting thing happened! Just before Christmas, 1974, we were home one night and turned the television on to watch a very special program. I SAW AN AMAZING THING! Would you like to know what I saw? I saw a great big fat "toad" on television — one of the most repulsive things that I had ever seen. I was fascinated by this big, fat ugly "toad," because she was very unique! Her voice sounded remarkably like mine, her husband's name was Charles, she was on a program called THE HAPPY HUNTERS and she had a dress on exactly like the one hanging in my closet.

I looked at this big fat "toad" and my heart cried out to God. I said, "God, how can you use a mess like me? How can you use anybody who is as revolting looking as I am?" My heart cried from the very depths of my soul! I cried out, "God, who would ever listen to me when I tell them that Jesus Christ is the answer to every problem in life, when I look like this." My heart continued to break. The more I watched the program, the more my heart broke, and I said, "Oh, God, I'm a mess! This problem is something I've wrestled with all of my life. And I have been a miserable failure where food is concerned. Lord, I can't do it, you'll have to do it! Show me what to do!" I WAS DESPERATE! (Isn't it interesting to note that years before I said the same thing about cigarettes.)

Shortly after this God began to put me in contact with some of my great Christian friends who all of a sudden had dropped a miraculous amount of weight. When I asked each one of them how they had lost, they all told me the same thing. "You ought to try HCG shots." My heart really cried out to God because I said, "God, I need to know what to do. I don't really think I know at this point what to eat and what not to eat. I just don't know where to start." I continued to cry out, "Lord, what shall I do?" I began to meet other Christian friends who had gone on HCG shots, and others, and others, and finally I said, "Lord are you trying to tell me to go to a doctor to get the information that I just plain don't have but that I desperately need?" God said, "Go to a doctor."

I especially love the second chapter of Proverbs in the Living Bible starting with the third verse. He says, "Yes, if you want better insight and discernment, and are searching for them as you would for lost money or hidden treasure, then wisdom will be given you, and knowledge of God himself; you will soon learn the importance of reverence for the Lord and of trusting him. For the Lord grants wisdom! His every word is a treasure of knowledge and understanding." I knew that some way God was telling me to keep on searching for the way and that he would give me the wisdom that I needed. The book of Proverbs also has a lot to say about common sense, and I think many times we fail to use the good common sense God has given concerning our eating habits.

Then, in God's beautiful plan, he made it possible for me to meet a very outstanding doctor in weight control, Dr. Paul McGuff. I went to him, explained my problem and told him that I was absolutely desperate. I want you to understand that I have prayed ever since I have been a Christian about my weight. It amazes me when I look back now to see that I had no problem giving up my cigarettes, I had no problem laying alcohol on the altar, I had no problem laying a polluted mouth on the altar, I had no problem laying a lot of other things on the altar. I guess because we know we have to eat something, we forget that we can put our appetite on the altar too!

I became aware of the fact that I didn't really know very much about food. As I said, I've been on every single solitary diet that you can imagine. As I thought about the different diets, I realized that I didn't really have ANY knowledge, I was just blindly following somebody else down a road and I had no knowledge whatsoever to back up what I was doing.

I took 33 blood tests to see what physical condition I was in because the doctor said he would not allow me to take the HCG and go on a very rigid fat free diet if I was not in good physical condition. I passed 32 with flying colors, but my triglyceride count was 428! The thing that really panicked me was when I discovered that all I could eat was 500 calories a day! *I could eat more than that in one "secret" snack!* I remember saying to the doctor, "I'll never be able to do it — NO WAY!!!"

I started taking HCG shots under Dr. McGuff's supervision. I'm not going to comment for or against the shots because God gave me a specific purpose in doing this. I do know this program taught me a discipline which I have never had before concerning food. God used this to give me my start in wisdom and knowledge for food. The only reason as a Christian that I was able to take them was because they do not contain anything to get you revved up, there's no barbituate or drug of any kind in them. It is a natural product and therefore I felt no reluctance about taking it. I also checked with our own family physician who is a Spirit-filled man. He said he could see nothing in the makeup of HCG that would be harmful in any way or that would go against any Christian principles. He did, however, make a very interesting statement. He said "I don't really believe that there's anything in it that will help you lose weight." After much prayer, Charles and I felt I should go ahead.

The more I thought about 500 calories, the more I knew it was impossible for me to exist on that small amount of food. But God had put such a desire in my heart to lose weight that I knew somehow or other he was going to be in the whole program. I cried out, "God, you've got to do it, because there's no way I can exist on 500 calories a day." I had made such a mess of my weight my whole life, so, I knew I needed a greater help than I could give myself. Someway in that moment I managed to say "Lord, I'll never make it, this will be just another one of those things that I have tried so many times over the years, unless you really help me."

I read what we could have to eat, and I thought to myself "There's no way I can get by on that little bit of food, there is ABSOLUTELY NO WAY." 500 calories is a ridiculously small amount of food, so I thought! To make matters really worse, the doctor said I should go on a complete fast the second day of the diet. The second day of the diet in my case was Christmas day! I had invited a number of people for Christmas dinner and I thought, "What am I doing to do now?" The Lord said, "Fast the whole day long." I said, "Lord, you've got to do it, you've got to do it! I'm doing this for you, you've got to really help me because I can't call these people and tell them I can't have them for Christmas dinner. I've got to go ahead and cook the dinner." I knew I couldn't smell all that good food without having to weaken and break my fast. Believe it or not, on the second day of my diet, I cooked a turkey and dressing with all the trimmings and God gave me such a supernatural discipline that I did not eat one single bite! He let me look at the food, smell it as I cooked it without being absolutely completely dissolved by fleshly desires to eat everything that was on the table.

I was really excited because I felt I had passed the first milestone. Then came the next day when I was privileged to eat. The suggested menu was a piece of fish for lunch.

The diet said I could have 3½ ounces. I got a little piece of fish out of our freezer to cook, but it was such a little piece of fish, I decided I had better weigh it to make sure it was a full 3½ ounces. I wanted to make sure I got every bite coming to me. (You can see my old carnal nature was still in there working, trying to get all the food possible.) I brought my postage scale into the kitchen, put the piece of fish on wax paper and weighed it, and you'll never guess what! It weighed 7¾ ounces! I looked at the most minute piece of fish I'd ever seen in my whole life and said, "God, you mean I can only have less than half of that?" Miraculously, however, God had put within my heart a desire to listen to what he was telling me about food, so I reluctantly cut that tiny little piece of fish in half, weighed it again, cut off another little sliver, until it weighed exactly 3½ ounces before I stuck it in the broiler.

One thing this thoroughly convinced me of was to appreciate every tiny little bite. But I was still operating in the flesh, wanting every bite! God gave me tremendous discipline, a discipline I've never had in my entire life with food, and even though we were traveling I managed to stay on the diet. I took canned shrimp and canned fish along with me. We ate in hotel or motel rooms instead of dining rooms, and if you don't think it is difficult to pass by a delightful smorgasbord buffet with all the fantastic food on it that you love, and walk up to your room and eat a can of cold salmon, think again! There is no way you can do something like this in the flesh. It has to be God! Somehow or other it wasn't difficult because I kept screaming out to God, "God, you've got to do it, I just simply cannot."

Days went on and I began to discover that I was enjoying the fish, and meat didn't look nearly as good as it used to look. Those steaks that once looked so fabulous didn't appeal to me any more. It seemed I was taking a tremendous delight in fish, but it really wasn't that. Actually I was taking a tremendous delight in the Lord and I was just thanking him and praising him for what he was doing. By the time summertime came around, I had lost over 40 pounds. I had to have 7 inches taken out of my dresses, and I was absolutely thrilled with what God had done. The fat free diet brought my triglyceride count down to a normal 84. *What I had thought to be a tremendous tumor in my stomach turned out to be nothing but plain fat!* It miraculously began to disappear!

The time came to go off the shots with the recommendation that I stay on a maintenance diet to control my weight. Guess what happened? I was still operating in the flesh, and that old nature came right back in and I rewarded myself with a beautiful piece of gooey pastry because I had lost so much weight! Hallelujah! What a way to reward a dieter! Absolutely marvelous reward for all my discipline! (Stupid, but typical, wasn't it?) The thing that I had missed the most during the diet was a sweet roll for breakfast, so I decided to stay on a maintenance diet, but give myself a "reward" of a sweet roll for breakfast. One sweet roll wouldn't have been bad, but then the second one came and pretty soon it seemed we managed to have a sweet roll at night before we went to bed and a sweet roll for breakfast. I'd eat fish the rest of the day, but you see I was still lying to myself. I was still saying "I can hold my weight and eat these things that I know are going to put on weight." That's the same thing an alcoholic says when he takes one drink! Why do we try to kid ourselves?

Before the end of summer I had gained back close to 10 pounds. I really panicked but I was powerless to do anything about it! I said, "Lord, I don't want this. Is it going to be the same thing all over again? Am I a hopeless mess that never has the opportunity to stay thin without denying myself food all the days of my life?" Over and over again I cried out and said, "God, you made the good food that's on this earth and I know that you intend for us

to eat it or you would never have made it. But why is it
that all I have to do is look at something and I begin
to get desires again. My desires never stay under your
control!"

Right in the midst of all this turmoil about how fast I
was going to gain the weight back, God gave me the most
tremendous burden for overweight Christians. How
could I help anyone else when I was slipping right back
into my old eating habits? One thing I learned was YOU
CANNOT GO BACK TO YOUR OLD EATING HABITS!

God gave me the answer in a most interesting and
unique way while I was giving a talk on "God's Part and
Our Part." I was in the 4th Chapter of Ephesians at the 25th
verse and I read "Stop lying to each other; tell the truth,
for we are parts of each other and when we lie to each
other we are hurting ourselves." I said, "Christians don't
lie, do they? . . . or do they?" I was going to talk about the
Christians who speed and watch the rear view mirror and
pray they don't get caught! In the pause I made after "or
do they?" God spoke very loud and clear and I almost fell
off the rostrum. He said "Fat Christians are the biggest
liars of them all — and you're a FAT Christian." Ouch!
That hurt, but I began to think quickly about what he had
said and I realized it was true!

I stood there and realized how many times I've said
I must have some kind of a glandular problem. That's not
true at all! My thyroid was destroyed years ago, and yet
God has rebuilt it in the last 10 years and it functions
perfectly normal! I had no glandular problem, that was
just an excuse, and not a very truthful excuse at that.
Did you ever use the same one? I stood right in that
pulpit and shared what God had said to me and for the
first time in my life I said "I AM A FOODAHOLIC!" I
couldn't believe I had said it!

I believe that the temptation to overeat will always be
there. I really cried out to God. I cried over and over and

over again, and said, "God, I am a plain old foodaholic. I DO NOT UNDERSTAND IT. I have given everything else to you, but somehow or another I cannot give this to you."

As I write this book I can also see that God did a tremendous thing. HE MADE ME GET COMPLETELY HONEST WITH MYSELF FIRST OF ALL. He made me admit that I am a foodaholic. I believe a foodaholic is exactly like an alcoholic. We have to admit the problem to ourselves and be very honest about it. I often think how many times I said I could just look at a hot fudge sundae and gain weight. That isn't true at all. I wouldn't gain an ounce if I just looked at it. But my problem was I wanted to eat it. AND I DID EAT IT. I remember many times I have said I can just breathe air and gain weight. That isn't true at all. A foodaholic has to be perfectly honest and say, "I am fat BECAUSE I EAT TOO MUCH!" The doctor that God sent me to has a beautiful sign on his wall that says, "Don't wail on the scale if you cheat when you eat." I think this is one of the most fantastic things I've ever heard because it is the truth. The reason we wail when we get on the scale is because we have cheated or lied about the amount of food we eat.

I felt trapped, because God had called on me now to minister to the foodaholic and how could I help them when I couldn't get victory in my own life where weight was concerned. At one time there was a part of me that loved to drink martinis. I had no difficulty giving him this. There was a part of me that loved cigarettes. I loved them so much I smoked five packs every day, yet I didn't find this difficult at all because God really convicted me that my body was not a holy temple as long as I was smoking cigarettes. I had no problem giving him this, but somehow or other God never got through to me concerning food the fact that my body was "the holy temple of God and him who defiles it I will destroy." I could apply this to martinis, I could apply it to an alcoholic, I could apply it to cigarettes; and yet I could not apply it to food. Suddenly I began to see that my body was the holy temple of God and that by defiling it with an excess amount of food, God was going to let me destroy myself. I heard Graham Kerr (the Galloping Gourmet) make a statement that as much as 25% of your life can be cut off by overweight. I thought, "I'm getting old enough that, if I cut off 25% of my life, I won't have much left." I think we all have the same natural instinct to preserve ourselves.

I believe God looked deep into my heart and saw that for the first time in my entire life I was going to be willing to give him that part of me that really loves to eat. He let me gain another half pound, then another half pound . . . and ANOTHER! I saw I was on exactly the same dead end street I had traveled BEFORE! Was this going to be a repeat performance? WAS THERE NO ANSWER? I knew that I had lost weight by cutting down calories, but who wants to starve their entire life long? Was that the only answer? I couldn't do it. I LOVE TO EAT! I LOVE TO EAT ALL KINDS OF FATTENING FOOD! I COULDN'T GO WITHOUT THEM THE REST OF MY LIFE. I'D BE MISERABLE!!! Suddenly, it was like a bolt of lightening I DIDN'T CARE whether I did or not! I was that desperate! I wanted to be somebody God could use! I had prayed for years, "God, get rid of this fat, get rid of this fat." I had given him my weight for years, but I became aware of the fact that my weight was not the problem, IT WAS MY APPETITE!! Finally, in sheer desperation, I cried out in some of the greatest agony I have ever known, "God, if I never get to eat another rich gooey pastry the rest of my life, I'll do it for you. GOD, IF I NEVER GET TO EAT ANOTHER THING THAT I REALLY LOVE, I'LL DO IT FOR YOU. I GIVE YOU MY APPETITE!

With that simple little decision of my own will, God did a miracle! HE COMPLETELY TOOK AWAY MY DESIRE

FOR FOOD!
It was that simple!

CHAPTER III

HOW DID IT START
AND WHERE DOES IT END?

"Take delight in the Lord, and he will give you the desires of your heart." Psalm 37:4 (RSV)

God has a very exciting way of watching over us even when we're tiny little children. Even as small children there were times when we prayed prayers that we didn't really mean, if we had sat down to think about what the end result was going to be. The following is typical.

My parents were very poor! As a matter of fact, I remember when we were very small children, my mother and daddy and my older sister and I lived in one dingy furnished room somewhere in a not-too-elegant area of Chicago. It was just after a stock market crash, and the tiny bit of money that my daddy had hoped to spiral into a fortune, so that he could give his family everything they wanted, all of a sudden was wiped out and everything we had was gone, even though it wasn't very much to begin with.

I remember, even though I was a very tiny little child, living in this miserable little room. I can still see it today in my mind and would recognize the room if I walked into it. The thing that I can see the plainest is a bag of potatoes sitting in the corner . . . a great BIG bag of potatoes. Do you know why I remember that bag of potatoes so well? Because that was all we had to eat! That one big bag of potatoes had to feed us for every single meal. We had boiled potatoes for breakfast, we had boiled potatoes for lunch, and we had boiled potatoes for supper.

If we would look back upon some of the things that happened to us many, many years ago, a lot of us might be able to find out where the desire for overeating started. I have a feeling mine might have started right there, because I hated potatoes. Not only did I hate them, I thoroughly despised potatoes, and the idea of having potatoes three times a day was the most miserable thing in the world I could think of. Yet that was all we had to eat, boiled potatoes morning, noon and night. I don't know if the desire to eat came into my heart at that exact time or if I was too little then to actually remember very much about it; but I do know by the time I was old enough to go to school, I had an obsession for food. One of the things that we never had any money for was milk. Day after day in school I'd see the kids bring two pennies in to buy a little half pint bottle of milk. How I envied them! I always thought the most wonderful thing in the world would be to have enough money to buy a little tiny bottle of cold milk, but the money was never there. My mother got sick with tuberculosis when we were small, my daddy had to put her in the sanitarium, so there was even less money. It seemed to me we ate potatoes, ATE POTATOES, ATE POTATOES for an awful long time.

At this time ice cream parlors were very popular. The funny kind that had the little fancy stools. If you weighed very much and you sat on them, you'd break them down! Yet, it always seemed to me that they had the most elegant looking things in these funny, little bitty stores. I remember standing outside the window because I never had enough money to go in and buy anything, and looking at the beautiful concoctions they made of ice cream and bananas and nuts and cherries and whipped cream. I remember thinking to myself, "When I get old enough I'm going to have enough money *so I can buy a banana split every single day of my life.*" As a hungry little kid, who didn't even know what ice cream tasted like, there was planted within my heart a desire to be able to eat everything that I possibly could. Somewhere in those young years, I guess, there came this fervent desire to be rich and successful some day for just one reason — SO THAT I COULD HAVE ALL THE FOOD I WANTED TO EAT!

I wonder today what the store owner must have thought about this skinny little girl who finally got up enough courage to come in there and just look, but with never any money to buy. I remember I'd stand there and watch them as they'd make ice cream cones for other people. It always fascinated me how they could dip the ice cream cone into chocolate and then the chocolate would instantly freeze before they handed out this delicacy to somebody other than me. I remember also that I'd get around on the side so that I could look in and see all these sparkling little things they used to call rainbow cones. They would put vanilla ice cream on a cone, and then they would roll it around in multi-colored sparkles — red, green, yellow, orange, blue, purple. It made the most interesting and exciting looking thing in the world. Someday, I thought, I'll be able to eat all of that I want! I'm going to work so hard when I grow up that I will have all the money I want, so I can eat all of the ice cream that I want. I'll eat a banana split every day, and when I have children I'm going to let them eat all the ice cream they want!

Maybe this is where it started. I really don't know, but I do know that weight has been a problem my entire life. *I've probably lost 20,000 pounds in my entire life, and successfully gained it all back again.* My skin, I've often felt, is like rubber. I'm either fat like a BIG rubber ball, or skinny for a little while like a rubber band. I hate to say it, but most of the time I've been like that fat beach ball that looked so tight it was about to burst at any moment. I sometimes wonder if what I was saying at that time about being so rich that I could afford a banana split, wasn't really a prayer to God, that I was saying, "God, let me make enough money so I can afford to eat the kind of food I THINK I'd like to eat."

If I had known what I was really praying, I would never have asked that, because who can eat banana splits every day of their life? In the first place, I think they'd get to the point where they wouldn't taste very good, would they? Then think of the devastating effect they can have on your figure and upon your health.

While my mother was in the tuberculosis sanitarium I decided also that I was going to be a good cook. One day, when my daddy was away, my sister, who is just twenty months older than I, and I decided we were going to cook oatmeal. Because of the tremendous hunger I had within my little heart for everything I could possibly get, we decided to cook a whole box! We started with one pan, then we had to pour it into another pan because it started growing. Soon we had to pour it into a third pan because it kept growing, and then a fourth and a fifth. Pretty soon we had every pot in the house and every bowl full of half-cooked oatmeal. We eventually ate it, because I have a sneaky feeling my father punished us for making such a mess of things by making us eat it!

One of the things Daddy always said was, "Clean your plate. We can't afford to waste anything." So instead of throwing something away when we'd eaten all we wanted, we proceeded to keep eating until our plates were clean.

My mother eventually came home from the hospital and we relinquished most of the household duties, since we were at this time about seven and eight years old. Most children are really impressed with their mother's cooking, but for some reason or another, I never was. I say this with all due respect to my mother because she made the best chicken and dumplings in the entire world, and she also made the best cherry pie. But that was about the only thing she ever learned to cook. I made up my mind I was going to learn to be the best cook in the world! My mother was a very plain cook, and maybe that's why I didn't like her food. I wanted rich stuff. I wanted stuff gobbed up with whipped cream! I wanted her to make rich, brown gravy with every single meal, because somehow in my heart I associated brown gravy with rich people. I thought only rich people could eat brown gravy and that poor people could not. At that time we had fried chicken and milk gravy, but to me that was "country" gravy. I wanted this rich, brown gravy that I had seen in a restaurant one time that people poured on top of mashed potatoes, and it looked so good. My little taste buds were just dying to try it, but it was years before I ever did.

Watch at what an early age little lies came in about food! Food had gotten to be something that was super important in my life, because we just didn't have enough. Food became a god I didn't have. We used to take a ride on Sunday afternoons. It was THE THING to whiz around the country in a Model T Ford, going probably all of twenty miles on a Sunday afternoon, because you couldn't go fast enough to go further than that. We couldn't afford to eat out, so we'd have to take a sandwich or picnic lunch along. Somehow we always managed to wheedle our daddy into stopping at a filling station and we would get a candy bar.

At that time there was a candy bar called "Chicken Dinner." I'd go to school the next day, and in an effort to impress my little friends with the fact that we really ate good, I would say, "We went for a ride yesterday and stopped at this real nice place, and we had a chicken dinner!" Well, we really did have a "Chicken Dinner" but not what they were thinking about and not what I'd implied with my little tiny white lies about food.

When I was somewhere between nine and ten I was invited to a birthday party. I had never been to a party like this except once before in my life. I don't even remember what the first party was all about except that it was a birthday party, and everybody was really dressed up. But I do remember this girl's party, and I remember her name to this day. Do you know why? We had RED Koolade! I had never tasted Koolade in my entire life, because all we had to drink at our house was water. What a pig I made of myself! I MUST HAVE HAD AT LEAST TEN GLASSES! I just stood at the punch bowl, and as soon as they would fill my glass I would drink it and stand there with my little hand stuck out with my glass, my eyes saying, "May I have another glass, please?" Finally, the mother of the little girl who had the birthday party said, "Honey, haven't you ever tasted anything like this before?" I was so embarrassed because I had to admit that I had never tasted anything like that in my whole life. I never knew there was anything that good!

Over and over again I heard, "Clean your plate. Clean your plate." Once a week we had dessert, and we never got ours unless we had cleaned our plate every meal all week long. Whether we had more than we wanted or whether we had food we didn't want, or whether we had things that were fattening and not good for us, we had to eat it. We had to clean our plate because we were constantly told it was a sin to waste food. When I was good, I got dessert. When I was bad, I didn't. As a result, I grew up thinking that desserts were a reward for being good! I wonder how many of us have exactly the same hangup. Maybe we love sweets because we like to feel we are being rewarded for being good.

Candy was something that was unheard of in our house. I remember visiting other children's homes at Christmas and seeing candy all over the place, and yet in our house we just could not afford it.

My mother and daddy loved us in a very special way. Somehow, with mother having been sick ever since I was born, there just wasn't money left over. Everything we had had to go to pay doctor and hospital bills for her. All of these things, I guess, left a mark on me. I have not thought of most of them until I started to write this book. God has given me a tremendous burden for people who, like myself, have always had a problem with weight. Maybe you'll discover the reason for your overeating through the pages of this book.

We continued to clean our plates. When I look back now, I see we ate all the foods that were really wrong, because they were the cheap things to eat, but I had no weight problem then. Why? We didn't overeat! I carefully ate everything on my plate, because I didn't want to miss out on that one little bit of dessert we had at the end of each week. But we didn't get too much on our plates.

We grew a little more prosperous, and I remember somewhere along the line we used to get one pint of ice cream a week. Daddy had half of it. Mother had a fourth of it. My sister and I shared the last quarter between the two of us. I remember that I enjoyed it and dearly loved it and thought, "Someday, I'm going to have all the ice cream I want all the time."

Can you see how all of these circumstances were putting into my mind some permanent impressions about food? I often look at my own children, and I think of how many times I've said to them, "Would you like some ice cream for dessert?" The first question they asked me was, "What kind do we have?" So, I named three, four, or five kinds that were in the freezer, and they said, "Oh, I don't like that. Haven't you got something else?" I often wonder what I would have done if I had had my choice of all the flavors of ice cream I could possibly eat. I didn't, so all of these little things concerning food kept stockpiling.

My mother died shortly after I graduated from high
school. By this time I was working and making my own living. When I think of the salary I made at that time, it is absolutely hysterical, because it was so little in comparison
with what people make today. Yet, I suppose it did go just
as far or even farther.

I had been denied clothes all of my life, because that
was another one of the things we couldn't afford. I
remember in high school I had two dresses per year. Not
actually two dresses; I had one dress and one sweater
and one skirt, and that was all. One day I wore the dress
and the next day I wore the sweater and skirt. The next
day I wore the dress, and the next day I wore the sweater
and skirt. It didn't make any difference whether it was
Saturday, Sunday, Monday, Tuesday, Wednesday,
Thursday, or Friday. That was all I had. If I didn't grow
too much, I got to wear the same dress the next year; but
if I grew fast enough I got another new sweater and a new
skirt, and a new dress. Because my sister was older than
I and a little bit bigger, I remembered that sometimes I
got her hand-me-downs, so it was a long time in between
new dresses.

I'll never understand how we were so happy, but we
were. Still, within me there was this "thing" that really de-
veloped. This "thing" said, "Someday, I'm going to be rich
enough to buy and eat all the food I can hold."

After our mother died my sister and I lived by ourselves. I did the cooking. I did most of the shopping,
because I was the one who really loved to eat. Now, in
spite of not having clothes when I went to high school at
an age when every girl wants to really look her best, you
would have thought that my first interest would have
been to go out and buy clothes as soon as I got a job, but
it wasn't. *I spent my money for food!*

My sister and I lived in an apartment together, because our daddy was a traveling salesman who just came

home over the weekend, and the biggest fights we ever had were over the money I spent on food. We shared equally the expenses of the cost of living, including food. And, I remember the biggest hassles were because I always wanted to spend a lot of money on food, and she always wanted to very carefully measure out the money and buy just the exact amount of food that was necessary.

It's very interesting that while we were both brought up under the same circumstances, my sister has never had a problem with weight. Today she weighs about 120 pounds; and in order to maintain this, she has to force herself to eat some big delicacy every night, or her weight will go under 120 pounds.

But that tremendous desire was there, not only for food and a lot of it, but for good food. I began to buy cookbooks, I began learning how to cook, and I learned to make gravy! I learned how to cook macaroni and cheese. I learned how to make spaghetti. I learned how to make lasagna. I learned that baked potatoes were delicious with loads of sour cream, loads of butter, loads of grated cheese, and loads of bacon crumbled on top. I learned to make chicken curry, and on top of the chicken curry I would put all of the fattening things in the world you can think of! Toasted coconut, slivered almonds, home made chutney, bacon crumbles, grated egg, french fried onions, etc.! No wonder I had to have my gall bladder taken out before I was 45 years old!

I learned to make cakes, and I learned to make pies, but I never learned to make the kind of cakes that might have been acceptable on a diet. I learned to make the ones where you put fudge icing on top about half an inch thick. Then you made a fantastic fudge filling to go on the inside. Then you dribbled the frosting all over the place until you could eat it with a spoon. On top of this I loaded nuts and any other fattening thing I could think of! I always put nuts in the cake dough, nuts in between the cake and nuts on top of the cake. As a matter of fact, it looked almost like a solid nut cake.

When it came to pies, this was one of my real specialities. I never liked just the plain old pie dough for a crust. I liked a sweet crust, so I learned how to make the most fantastic graham cracker crust in the world. It had sugar and butter until it was so rich it would just fall apart and dissolve in your mouth. On the inside of this I always put the super-rich fillings, made not with milk but with cream and eggs and all the fattening things in the world you can think of. Chocolate was my real favorite, and I loved to put twice the amount of baking chocolate in a pie, just because I loved the real strong taste of dark chocolate. After the pie ended up to be about an inch and a half high, then I always loaded each pie with two cartons of whipped cream; so you can imagine what the pie looked like. Then, do you know what I did? I ate the biggest piece of all. I really *loved* to eat it. I always loved to give my guests lots of food, but then there was always plenty left over. After the company went home, if there was only one piece of this *huge* chocolate pie left, I ate it so I wouldn't have to put it in the refrigerator. There always was one left because I cut the pie into one more piece than we needed.

By this time I had married and had my first child, Tom. I thought in order to be a good mother I had to be the best cook in the world, so I began *cramming him full of all kinds of good, fattening things*.

I've always been a very gregarious person, and I love to have people around me. I felt that if I had people over for dinner this would show that I really loved them. If I had them over for dinner and gave them more than they could eat, I felt that this really was a tremendous indication of the love I had for them. We had company once or twice a week and we would always have a very elegant dinner. I would have everything you could think of and even more. I always cooked more than anybody needed, because I didn't want anyone to go away from my table hungry. I proudly stated that no one ever left my table hungry. Maybe miserable, but not hungry!

I had married into a German family, and my mother-in-law also loved to cook. A few years after marriage I began to notice that I was getting heavier and heavier and heavier, and the dresses got to be a larger size and a larger size and a larger size. In spite of the fact that my husband was ill, I still managed to be happy. Even though I wasn't a Christian, God blessed me and allowed me to make a living for our family and in his great love and mercy gave me a peace that took me through the circumstances of losing my mother, my father and my husband before I was 35.

My son and I moved to Florida when his daddy died and we began to make friends there whom we invited over for dinner. Florida is a magnificent place to have people for outdoor dinners, and one of the specialties I had was barbecued chicken. The chicken might not have been fattening, except that the barbecue sauce I made had two cups of brown sugar in it plus tomatoes, catsup, barbecue sauce, everything you could possibly think of and probably had a "thousand" calories per cup. The chicken was barbecued with this sauce drizzled all over it, then it was put back into the sauce so that it could just soak it up and be the most fattening thing in the world.

These were dinners where people brought food, and I remember a friend made some delightful things called squiggles, which is a fantastic Italian dish that was just loaded with calories, cheese, tomato paste, pasta, the whole works. We jubilantly rejoiced on the back porch every Sunday as we were having these magnificent meals. Within my heart I felt by giving people a tremendous amount of rich food I was really showing love. Little did I realize the damage I was doing to my own body as a result of this (not to mention theirs). I continued to eat more and more and more. I continued to get fatter and fatter and fatter.

Tom, Joan, and I went through some real traumatic experiences when all of a sudden there was a tremendous lack of money. I had just started a printing company with so little money it was unbelievable. I had every strike against me in the world. I was over the age where they say you can be a success in the business world. I was under-capitalized. I had two small children, and I was a woman. Somehow or another, God, in his love and his mercy, had his hand on me all throughout the years; I can see that now.

For a period of about six months I was again thrust back into the problem I had as a little child. There was no money to buy food. There was no food, and as hard as it is for me to imagine it today and to even tell it, would you like to know how I fed my children? There are many supermarkets which throw away the rotten vegetables and rotten fruit at night. They put this rotting produce in a trash can or garbage can, and anyone who wants to may come in and pick out what they want. Maybe it was pride, but there was no way I could bring myself to ask for welfare. Somehow or another I still believed that "I" was capable of bringing my family out of this dilemma.

For a period of six months we lived on three dollars a week grocery money. When I look back now, I don't know how we did it, but I remember the food was little and far between. I'd give Tom two eggs every morning. Joan, being younger, would get one egg and I got one egg. Each one of them got a little money for lunch because they were both in school. Joan was in a private school and Tom in a public school. I had nothing left for lunch. Then came supper and it was the same routine again, two eggs for Tom because he was bigger, one egg for Joan, and one for me. In a period of less than three months I lost fifty pounds; and this should have told me at that time that my whole problem was overeating, but all it did was to increase my desire to be a success so I could buy enough food that we could have all we wanted to eat.

I remember standing there many nights until midnight peeling fruits and vegetables and cutting away the rotten parts. Maybe out of one whole peach there would be just one bite that was worth eating. This was the only way my children could have any of the little luxuries like fresh fruit or an occasional fresh vegetable. I remember praying to God, even though I wasn't a Christian, and asking him to let me be a success so I could give my children all the food they wanted. It amazes me even more that God was somehow real enough to me that I didn't "wish," but I "prayed."

Time passed and God blessed my business. I guess he knew what was going to happen to me eventually. So, he blessed me and I began to make enough money. What was the first thing I spent it for? Clothes? *No, I spent it for food.* Once again I was back to that same problem I had as a little girl, wanting to eat and eat and eat. And eat and eat, we did. I remember that Joanie as a little tiny girl was so thin that my mother-in-law said, "You'll never raise her. She's so delicate and fragile." So, I would cram food into her. I'd say, "Eat it. Eat it. It's good for you." I think that one of the injustices mothers do to their children is to say, "Eat it. Eat it. Think how many poor little children in China don't have anything to eat. Think of all the hungry little children there are in India. Think of all the hungry little children here, and you don't want to eat it. Eat it right now." I have a compassion for underfed people, but our eating excessively doesn't help them. What good does it do the wonderful Chinese for you to clean your plate?

I had to go to work, so I started a printing company when Joan was very young. Bless her little heart, she spent most of her growing-up years in the back of a print shop. I had a little cot where I could put her, but most of the time she slept on a blanket on the floor when she got too tired to sit up any longer. I had to make up somehow or another for the fact that I was working such long hours and keeping her up long after she should have been in bed. Her prize for always being such a good girl was an extra pizza or maybe it was a double-dip ice cream cone from the ice cream store on the corner. So, Joan, because of the lack of time I could give her like a mother should, began to look upon pizzas and French fried potatoes and ice cream sundaes, especially hot fudge ones with nuts on them, as a reward for being a good child. Joan has never been a problem in her entire life, but I can see now the effect of what I did to her at that time.

If ever I had a message for any mother, I would say, don't force your children to eat. Don't reward them for being good by giving them food, expecially by saying, "Eat your dinner or you can't have your dessert." You see, this puts desserts into that real ethereal realm of that special something you can have as a reward. Unfortunately, many people are going to go to their graves thinking that dessert is that super-special somethingyou get only when you are good. So we can sit and pat ourselves on the back and say, "See, I've been good. I had dessert today. I made chocolate cup cakes and put nuts and coconut and fudge frosting all over the top of them yesterday. This means that I'm good because I can eat sweet things like this, and the more I eat, the better I must have been."

Do you see what you're doing to yourself and your children when you do this? I really believe that there is a happy medium when children can be given dessert just as normally as they can be given vegetables. I believe that children generally have a little built-in system for eating the right foods if we don't try and cram them full of wrong ones. I also believe we need wisdom and knowledge to provide balanced, tasty, appetizing right kinds of food. Certainly discipline is essential but we have a responsibility to teach our children, as well as ourselves when, what

and how much to eat. We should have them well estab-
lished in a good eating pattern at an early age.

Milk has always been a "must" at my house. I guess
it's because I remember subconsciously that little girl in
school who looked so longingly at those other kids who
had a half pint of milk with a straw in it, that I decided my
kids would always have all the milk they wanted. So, I or-
dered milk by the gallon and said, "Drink it, drink it, drink
it, it's good for you. It'll make you strong, and it'll make
you healthy, it'll give you good teeth, it'll do this. It will do
that." And it will do all those things, BUT TOO MUCH
CAN ALSO PUT ON WEIGHT! So my kids grew big and
strong and healthier by the day — especially big!

Tom, being a boy, burned up his fat much quicker and
has never really had a problem except when he was
somewhere around 13 or 14. That's when Joan really
started. By the time she got to be 13 she weighed 185
pounds and has had a battle ever since. Do I blame Joan?
No, I do not. I take the blame totally and completely upon
myself, because I started her on bad eating habits. The
reason I'm being so completely honest with you and telling you about this is because I believe it might help you to
search out why you like to eat. I believe there's a reason
behind all of this, and I don't believe that God can really
help us in retraining our appetites until we are honest with
ourselves and admit why we like food.

One Christian lady said to me, "A Christian way to kill
yourself is to overeat, because you don't know how else to
get out of your problem in a Christian sort of way." She
said, "Think about it. The more I don't want to admit it the
more I feel this might be a part of my problem." Do we
sometimes so completely forget to give it all to God and
say, "God, it's too big for me, you handle it," that we
forget that Jesus is the answer. Overeating never helps any
problem; it only aggravates and accentuates that problem.

CHAPTER IV

WISDOM AND KNOWLEDGE
COME GALLOPING IN!

God brought the Galloping Gourmet into our lives at a very appropriate time. This man probably has as great a knowledge of food, the preparation of food, the caloric content and the nutritive value of food as any other person in the entire world. I began to share with him some of my problems in dieting and my concern for fat people. Graham had just become a Christian and had discovered the same thing as I — that there are an awful lot of fat Christians around.

I began to pick his brains for any and all advice he could give me as an individual and also something that I could share with other people. One of the first things he suggested that I do was to write to the United States Government Printing Office in Washington, D.C., for U.S.D.A. Handbook #8, and also for pamphlet #72, which give the nutritive values of foods. I sent for these right away! Graham said there are three things you need: WISDOM, KNOWLEDGE AND OBEDIENCE. Knowledge is available from sources such as these pamphlets, good books written by knowledgeable people who have learned through study, research, experiments and experience, from cookbooks, etc. Wisdom is attained by thinking, learning and applying knowledge, and it is attainable by anyone who has a normal mind and who wants to learn.

All the wisdom and knowledge in the world won't do us a bit of good unless we are obedient. This is where we really have to pray and ask God to help us be obedient (and we have to do *our* part). Then we have to be obedient when the Holy Spirit slaps our hand and says, "Get your hand out of that cookie jar," or when the Holy Spirit says, "Put that chocolate donut down because it is super fattening." Wisdom and knowledge, yes, but obedience to the voice of the Holy Spirit is the most important of all!

I began occasionally sharing a little information about some of the delightful ways I have learned to cook food, and to encourage people to lose weight. Almost every time I have spoken about fat, I have asked all who are at least 5 pounds overweight to stand. A minimum of 80% of the people stand as being 5 pounds or more overweight! Each one indicates a very sincere desire to lose weight and yet they have not had the discipline that is necessary.

The first time I ever shared on this subject at our monthly miracle service, 440 individuals turned in prayer cards indicating a total overweight of 15,485 pounds, or an average of 35+ pounds per person. A grand total of 7.3 tons. Would you believe it? I am sure that God in his sovereign way could just look at each one of us and say "be gone" and every ounce of excess fat we have on us would disappear, but I don't believe we would learn a thing by this. This is why I believe God allows us to read his word, to feast upon his word and then to quit feasting upon all these super delicacies. God doesn't forgive sin in our lives so we can fill ourselves up with sin again, and he's not going to "melt" the fat off of our bodies just so we can continue eating in a sinful way. We'd all like to be "Fat today and gone tomorrow," but that's not God's plan so I say "LOØSE IT" . . . Loose the bondage of self appeasement and the fat will go. Loose the power of God in you

life and give him your appetite. Loose it and lose it — for
Jesus!

As soon as I got the booklet on the nutritive values of
food I began to search for knowledge. I probably spent
three hours the day I received the booklet discovering the
caloric values of a lot of different foods. What a revelation!
I was never so shocked in my entire life! Some of the foods
I had always heard about for weight reducing diets
seemed to me to contain the most calories.

About this time I decided to really start watching my
caloric intake to see what would happen. I came up with a
new motto, and I hope you'll make this yours, too!
"JESUS, HOW LITTLE CAN I GET BY WITH — NOT HOW
MUCH CAN I EAT!" Have you ever been trapped by a diet
which says how MUCH you can eat? All you want — and
MORE! I have been on every kind of diet that insists you
can eat a tremendous amount of food, but it never worked
for me! With all my heart and soul I believe that a calorie is
a calorie, is a calorie, is a calorie — regardless of how or
when you eat that calorie. I don't believe there is any way
you can gorge yourself and still lose weight.

I began searching for truths concerning foods, and
decided it would really be fun to see how little I could get
by on. And would you like to know I discovered I can get
by on an amazingly small amount of food? Why . . . because I HAD GIVEN GOD MY APPETITE FOR THE FIRST
TIME IN MY LIFE — I HAD LAID MY DESIRE FOR FOOD
ON THE ALTAR! When you really mean business with God
and are willing to obey him, and you sincerely ask him to
take away your appetite, he will do it! There is no doubt in
my mind whatsoever that he will, but it isn't a question of
kidding God and kidding yourself. It's just a question of
honestly being willing to lay your appetite on the altar of
God, and leave it there!

I was sharing in Ohio and it seemed to me as though
200 of the 300 there weighed over 200 pounds. I never

saw so many fat women in my entire life, all of whose hearts were crying out to lose weight, and my heart was crying right with them! I shared the motto with them of "JESUS, HOW LITTLE CAN I GET BY WITH, NOT HOW MUCH CAN I EAT." I believe this could be the secret of YOUR weight loss, if you really mean it.

After our last service a young lady whom I do not even know came over and handed me a little piece of paper. She said, "Did you ever read what it says in Daniel about food?" I have read the book of Daniel many times, but I never really looked upon it in relation to weight control. The little slip of paper told me the verses to read. It was Daniel the first chapter from the eighth through the seventeenth verses:

8 But Daniel made up his mind not to eat the food and wine given to them by the king. He asked the superintendent for permission to eat other things instead. 9 Now as it happened, God had given the superintendent a special appreciation for Daniel, and sympathy for his predicament. 10 But he was alarmed by Daniel's suggestion.

"I'm afraid you will become pale and thin compared with the other youths your age," he said, "and then the king will behead me for neglecting my responsibilities."

11 Daniel talked it over with the steward who was appointed by the superintendent to look after Daniel, Hananiah, Misha-el, and Azariah, 12 and suggested a ten-day diet of only vegetables and water; 13 then, at the end of this trial period the steward could see how they looked in comparison with the other fellows who ate the king's rich food, and decide whether or not to let them continue their diet.

14 The steward finally agreed to the test. 15 Well, at the end of the ten days, Daniel and his three friends looked healthier and better nourished than the youths who had been eating the food supplied by the king! 16 So after that the steward fed them only vegetables and water, without the rich foods and wines!

17 God gave these four youths great ability to learn and they soon mastered all the literature and

science of the time, and God gave to Daniel special ability in understanding the meanings of
dreams and visions.

When I first read this in Daniel with weight control in
mind, God spoke to me about a Daniel "fast" and said,
"This is what I want you to go on." I really had difficulty in
the King James version, because it says, "And at the end of
ten days, their countenances appeared fairer and *fatter* in
flesh than all the children which did eat the portion of the
king's meat." I had a real problem with that word, "fatter,"
because I thought, "Well, if you're going to go on a
"Daniel fast" with the idea in mind of losing weight, who
wants to be fatter when you finish than you were at the
start?" I said, "Lord, surely you must have a better meaning." I continued to look in other King James versions, and
in the new Open Bible there was a little note defining fatter as "better looking." I decided to look a little further
and see what the Hebrew meaning was.

There are many different words or definitions in
Hebrew for the word "fat." Most of the times when it is
used in the Bible, it does mean "fat" as we think of it but
it also means an "anointing." The word "fat" means "to be
anointed, satisfied, rich or fertile." Now look back at this
and see what it says. And at the end of ten days, their
countenances appeared fairer and "more anointed" in the
flesh. They were more anointed, not necessarily fatter in
flesh, but more anointed by the Spirit of God, than all the
children which did eat the portion of the king's meat.

Drop down to the 17th verse. It says, As for these
four children, God gave them knowledge and skill in all
learning and wisdom. You see, they were anointed by
God to be smarter, to have more wisdom and knowledge
than they'd ever had in their entire life. All I can say is
"Thank you, Jesus." If this is going to do anything in my
life in this area, I am grateful for it.

This said the most interesting thing to me — a ten-day
diet of only vegetables and water. I thought, "Oh, how

gross! How absolutely awful — just plain old vegetables and water with no meat or butter for seasoning." Then I remembered all the delicious recipes I had cooked over the past few months without using any fat in the diet whatsoever. You see, it was my mind and my *attitude* that was changing. I began to THINK in the right direction. The devil loves to get hold of your mind and tell you can't do it, but all of a sudden I thought, "I think I'll try it." And God said, "I'm finally beginning to get through to you." I talked to Charles, and it was very exciting all of a sudden how we were aware that God was saying to start it off this way. We decided it was really a "Daniel fast" rather than a diet, because it was done in obedience to God and for his glory.

We started the fast — vegetables and water. The first thing I did was to get the wisdom and the knowledge I needed. I went to the charts and discovered all sorts of interesting things about vegetables. I had always heard that potatoes were a real "no-no" on any kind of weight-reduction diet. I discovered potatoes really aren't high in calories, provided you don't gob them up with butter, sour cream, bacon bits, grated cheese, and all those other little goodies we like to put on top of them.

I also made another amazing discovery. Baked potatoes plain are one of the most delicious foods in the world. I said to Charles, "What do we eat for breakfast, when all we're going to eat is vegetables? Who wakes up in the morning and wants to eat beets? Who wakes up in the morning and wants to eat an ear of corn? Not me! Who wakes up in the morning and wants to eat okra? Ugh! Who wants to wake up in the morning and eat asparagus?" But I said, "Lord, if these guys in Daniel got so much smarter and so much healthier and they got so much better looking at the end of ten days by eating just vegetables and water, then surely you can make us learn to like vegetables for breakfast."

We looked at all of the vegetables to decide which

one we thought would be best, and we decided on baked potatoes and mushrooms for breakfast. The first morning we got up and baked the potato, measuring it very carefully so we'd know exactly how many calories we were eating. We kept a chart so we knew exactly how many calories went into our body during the day. On top of the baked potato we had a half cup of mushrooms apiece. I had sauteed the mushrooms in soy sauce and water, and the potato was absolutely delicious with the addition of mushrooms. Excellent! fantastic!! We put seasoning salt on the potato before we baked it, and I said, "Charles, I think potatoes are absolutely fantastic for breakfast." Who ever heard of eating baked potatoes on a diet, and eating them for breakfast, of all things? This started us on a wild experiment to see how many exciting and different things we could have to eat, because the main problem with a diet is that it can be monotonous.

The most amazing thing happened when it came lunchtime. We looked at each other and said, "I can't eat anything, can you?" Neither one of us could eat a single solitary bite for lunch! We weren't hungry. We skipped lunch. About seven o'clock the first night we decided we'd better eat something again. But a peculiar thing had happened to both of us. Neither of us really felt the least bit hungry, so we put another little potato in the oven and ate it. Along with that I cooked one of our very favorites since I've been dieting. I cooked (stir-fried) cabbage, celery and onions for just a few moments in a little soy sauce and water and sprinkled lemon pepper on it; while it was still crisp and chewy we ate it. One cup of this was only 45 calories. With it we ate our potato. That was supper! The peculiar thing is that on this "Daniel fast" we had absolutely no hunger whatsoever. Both of us were feeling fantastic. We got up the next morning and decided we'd have another baked potato for breakfast, because we had enjoyed the one the

morning before so much. I cooked another cup of mushrooms, and we each had one half cup. We discovered a
repeat performance of the day before. When lunch time
came neither one of us could eat! *We weren't hungry.* Hallelujah, what a way to diet!

Suppertime came and again we had some celery, onions, and cabbage stir fried together. We also had one cup
of cooked tomatoes apiece. We were amazed to discover
for the first two days I had eaten under 400 calories each
day, which is almost unbelievable, because neither one of
us was the least bit hungry. The "Daniel fast" began to get
exciting. We decided to see how much variety we could
really put into our meals and have a great time and not get
bored. The next day we still stayed with the potatoes and
mushrooms for breakfast, because it was such a completely satisfying meal. We didn't realize we were being
loosed from the bondage of three meals a day. We were
discovering another part of God's answer to fat — loøse it!

We branched out for supper. We had a half cup of
beets and a big salad. We had a fourth of a head of lettuce,
a small tomato, cucumber slices, and a little green onion.
To our amazement my calories for the day added up to
only 422! AND WE HADN'T BEEN HUNGRY!! Anybody can
lose weight on that few calories. Along with our meals we
also drank hot tea. Hot tea seems to send a sensation to
your brain that your stomach has had food, whereas coffee seems to say "I'm hungry." Be sure to use a decaffein-
ated tea so you won't get "light headed."

Then came day number four and we were surprised to
discover that an ear of corn isn't too fattening. It doesn't
have any more calories than an apple, except when you
smear butter all over it. We had a huge salad, an ear of
sweet corn and a baked potato. We had a fantastic time,
because we were really making the Daniel fast an exciting
game for the Lord. What we really felt was that God was
teaching us something we could share with other people

who have the same problem as I. Our attitudes were fabulous — no griping, no complaining!

I want you to know that I really appreciate my husband Charles in this experiment. He has been willing to cooperate with me 100%, and I am well aware of the fact that there are many husbands who are not willing to go along with their wives. Charles does not have a weight problem and has never had a weight problem; yet he decided to see what would happen to someone who didn't need to lose weight if they went on this fast. Well, you might guess it. The very first thing that happened was that *Charles lost three pounds, and I lost nothing!* Now, you know, this can really be hard when you think, "Lord, what's the matter with me?" But, praise his holy name, the next day I dropped a pound and the next day another two pounds.

We decided while on the Daniel fast not to limit calories. In other words, our motto was, "Jesus, how little can I get by with, not how much can I eat." Peculiarly, the less we ate the less hungry we seemed to get.

You know there always has to be a real good testing period! Charles and I had been invited to a beautiful Chinese American church in Houston to help celebrate their nineteenth anniversary. They were having a banquet and asked us to be sure to come. Because they always have such fantastic Chinese food there, we declined, telling them that we were on this Daniel fast and really felt it was best that we not go around so much tempting food. We did tell them, however, that we would be glad to come and share in the anniversary.

When we arrived they were just starting to eat. Do you know what happens to your taste buds when all of a sudden you see this fantastic array of food? I love Chinese food, and I especially love it when it is made by the Chinese. It is just fantastic. I looked at this beautiful chop suey, and I looked at all the fabulous ways they cooked chicken. I looked at all the delicious fried rice. I looked at the bean sprouts. I looked at the mushrooms. I looked at the pork. I was shocked when I realized, "I'm not the least bit hungry." It had to be God! The temptation was there, and I really felt at this point that the devil was putting all of these fantastic foods in front of me, and yet there was no desire to eat anything whatsoever, because I had really given the problem to God! ". . . greater is he that is in you than he that is in the world." (I John 4:4 KJV). There is no temptation, even food, given to us that he will not give us the strength to overcome! We passed the first test with flying colors.

We were to leave the next day on a trip. We knew that we would have to break the fast, because there was no way we could get a baked potato for breakfast on a trip. We decided to take some of the chicken from the Chinese church home with us to eat when we broke the fast. Do you know what God did to us when we got home? He said, "Oh yes, you can keep on this Daniel fast while you are on this trip. You can take in your suitcase canned potatoes, canned tomatoes, canned asparagus, canned green beans, all those things that are low in calories. You put your butter salt in there and your seasoned salt and you can stay right on this fast the whole ten days. There is no excuse for you to go off just because you're going away to do my work." So, Charles and I packed in our suitcase canned potatoes, canned tomatoes, canned green beans, canned asparagus, and sat in the hotel and laughed and said, "I wonder if we thought years ago that we'd ever be sitting in a hotel room eating out of a can."

On a trip to Chicago, we had another real good testing. We have eaten many, many meals on planes. While many of them are very good, when you have the same menu over and over again it can get a little boring. We have flown (adding our miles together) over a million miles in the five and a half years since we've been married.

Now that we were on the Daniel fast, I had baked some potatoes just before we left the house, so we got on the plane carrying our baked potatoes. Then they brought the dinner.

We had decided we would take the meal so we could eat the salad they offered but nothing else. When they served the meal, we almost fell out of our seats. I don't believe I've ever seen such a delightful meal served on a plane. They served steak, a beautiful filet mignon that looked absolutely out of this world. They had almondine green beans, they had buttered carrots, they had carrot cake for dessert, loaded with nuts and frosting. Charles and I looked at it and absolutely had hysterics, especially when we looked at the gravy, which was loaded with mushrooms. "Satan, get thee behind me."

We took our little potatoes out of the sack; we ate the salad and had a cup of tea. Do you know that there was absolutely no regret in our hearts for not eating the steak, no desire whatsoever, because we knew that we were doing it for God. Having decided once and for all to give God my appetite, he saw to it that there was absolutely no problem involved.

Charles looked over at me and said, "You know what it really is, honey. You put your two desires down side by side. One is your desire for food, and the other is your desire for Jesus. Then, you choose which one you want." He continued, "Honey, I think you have finally made a decision you have postponed for years. *You have chosen Jesus over food!*" We really had a good Hallelujah time!

I'm going to ask you right now to do something. Put down two fingers, one from each hand. On the left side, say, "This is my desire for food. This is my desire that says, 'I can't live without all those sweet things, without all those goodies.' " Then, put the finger down on the right hand and say, "This is Jesus." Then, pick up the cross that you want to carry. I believe you'll choose Jesus. I don't believe there is any other choice for any of us but Jesus. The left hand will be too heavy to lift — but when the right hand comes up, the other will be "LEFT."

Would you turn to Proverbs 30 in the Living Bible? Starting with verse 7, "O God, I beg two favors from you before I die: First, help me never to tell a lie (about my weight or anything else). Second, give me neither poverty nor riches! Give me just enough to satisfy my needs!" *Give me just enough to satisfy my needs.* Isn't that a tremendous statement? "Jesus, how little can I get by with, not how much can I eat?" Said a little bit differently, but said in the word of God.

I'm going to ask you to right now turn to Psalms 145:15 in the Living Bible. It says, "The eyes of all mankind look up to you for help; you give them their food as they need it. You constantly satisfy the hunger and thirst of every living thing." You see, this is exactly what God did to us on the plane. He satisfied any appetite that we had, because we had given it to him. Had we stayed in the flesh, the steak would have looked and tasted good, the cake would have looked and tasted good, everything would have looked and tasted good. He satisfied our need with something as simple as a little tiny, unseasoned baked potato, just because we were doing it for him.

Verse 19 says, "He fulfills the desires of those who reverence and trust him." "Be delighted with the Lord. Then he will give you all your heart's desires." Psalm 37:4. Do you see how he changed the desires in our hearts? He gave us a desire to obey him, not the desires of our flesh, because peculiarly, I believe if we had eaten the steak and the carrot cake, the bread, and the butter, we would still not have been satisfied. Maybe momentarily our taste buds would have been satisfied; but our spirits would not have been satisfied, because we would not have reverenced and trusted God.

You'll notice there are many people who have fantastic ability at fasting; in other words, eating absolutely nothing. Somehow or another, when we use the word "diet" it sets up a reverberation in our mind that makes us want to rebel. I think it's because when we diet we think we are doing it for ourselves, and when we fast we are doing it for the Lord. That's why we've called this a "Daniel fast" rather than a "Daniel diet," because if you decide you'll do it for ten days, you'll do it for the Lord.

We made a very simple little chart from the U.S.D.A. Home and Garden Bulletin No. 72, and we want to show you just exactly the way we did it. We selected low calorie content vegetables. We're reproducing here some of the vegetables we and most people like the best and putting the caloric value by the side of each one. Then you can see also the amount of food we ate for days 1 through 10. You'll discover a chart for each of us, and the weight loss we attained. Charles acquired a virus and became quite ill at day seven (unrelated to the fast), so his covers only seven days. I lost eight pounds. Charles lost six.

We gave charts to interested people at our home Miracle Meeting. The average loss for the people who completed the Daniel fast was 8.38 pounds for 10 days. The highest loss was 13 pounds and only one person failed to lose anything. The average caloric intake for the 13 pound loser was 275½ per day! Accompanying the chart was a note: "Praise God for the 13 pounds plus! Through this experience I gave up drinking coffee. To him be the honor and glory forever." A 7 pound loser said "God gave me super willpower, something I haven't had." Another loser said "The diet was good. I plan to go on it again in 5 days or so!" Another 7 pound loser wrote a note "I feel great!" Several people did not complete the 10 day fast because in 5 days they lost the 5 pounds they had indicated they wanted to lose. Those who failed without a weight loss generally lost interest when they got hungry the first day, and did not continue beyond that. The man who showed no weight change averaged 1,024 calories per day. The others averaged only 393, believe it or not!

Charles just made a very interesting statement. He said, "Satisfying your stomach does not satisfy your whole being, but satisfying God satisfies your inner man and your entire being." I want you to think about that statement, because there is a lot of truth in it. If you're really serious about losing weight, you're going to have to give your appetite to God and let his power be loosed in your life. You loøsed your appetite to him and he will loose his power, and you will lose that unwanted extra burden of fat!

You might even want to go on a "Daniel fast." I would like to interject one word of caution here. If you were going on a fruit diet, you wouldn't eat all prunes, so be careful and don't select all of the "laxative" vegetables. These are the high roughage ones such as cabbage, celery, spinach, kale, leafy vegetables, etc.

50

NAME *Frances Hunter*

ADDRESS

CITY & STATE

10 Day Period Starting *10/1/75*

Weight at start: *171*

Weight at finish of 10 days: *162*

Tel. No.

Food (Vegetable)	Measure	Quantity	Weight	Calories	Day 1 Q	Day 1 C	Day 2 Q	Day 2 C	Day 3 Q	Day 3 C	Day 4 Q	Day 4 C	Day 5 Q	Day 5 C	Day 6 Q	Day 6 C	Day 7 Q	Day 7 C	Day 8 Q	Day 8 C	Day 9 Q	Day 9 C	Day 10 Q	Day 10 C
Soy sauce / Asparagus - Cooked	Cup	1		45		9		6		5		–	1	4 4	½	– 20		4		4 60				
Tea w/ saccharin / Green Beans, Cooked & Drained	*Cup* / Cup	1		*4* / 30	4	4			4	4	4	4	4	.	¼	4 7		4		4 13		10		
Beets, Canned or Cooked, Peeled	Cup	1		85					½	42					⅔	55	1	60						
Broccoli, Cooked, Drained	Cup	1		40													½	20						
Brussells Sprouts, Cooked	Cup	1		55																				
Cabbage, celery, onions / Cabbage, Raw, Shredded	*Cup* / Cup	*1* / 1		*45* / 15	1½	68	1	45	½	23			1	45										
Cooked	Cup	1		30																				
Carrots, Raw (5 1/2 x 1")	Ea	1		20					¼	5								10						
Cooked	Cup	1		45											¼	10								
Cauliflower, Cooked, Buds	Cup	1		25													2	100						
Celery, Raw (8¼x1½" at root end)	Stk	1		5				3						3			1	5						
Corn, Sweet, Ear 5 x 1 3/4"	Ea	1		70							1	70												
Cucumbers, 7½"x2"	Ea	1		30					⅙	5	⅙	5	⅙	5		5	1	30						
Lettuce, Iceberg, Raw 4-3/4"diam	Head	1		60					¼	15	¼	15	¼	15	⅛	8	¼	15		15		15		15
Mushrooms, Canned or boiled	Cup	1		40	½	20	½	20	½	20	½	20	½	20	½	20								
Okra, Cooked, Pods 3x 5/8"	Pods	8		25																				
Green onions / Onions, Cooked	Cup	1		60						3		3												
Popcorn / Peppers, Sweet, Raw or Cooked	Ea	1		15																				40 10
Potatoes, Baked or Boiled, Peeled	Oz.	1		17	7	119	8	136	6½	110	7½	128	5	85	4½ 5	78 85	6 8	102 136	1½	13	[illegible]	60 75		[illegible]
Radishes, Raw, Small	Ea	1		1																				
Sauerkraut, Canned	Cup	1		45																				
Spinach, Cooked *Soy*	Cup	1		45										15										
Squash, Summer, Cooked	Cup	1		30																				
Tomatoes, Raw, Diam. 3", 2-1/8"hg / Cooked	Cup / ea	1 / 1		50 / 40	1	50	1-	50	1	30 50	1	30	½	15	1	25	2	80	1	[illegible]		20		20
Total Calories Per Day					364		396		422 (~~377~~)		403		358		317		613		160		195		259	
Weight Loss Per Day					0		0		0		1		2		0		✓		✓		1			?

51

NAME *Charles Hunter* — 10 Day Period Starting *10-1-75*

ADDRESS ______ — Weight at start: *171*

Weight at finish of 10 days: *165*

CITY & STATE ______ — Tel. No. ______

Food (Vegetable)	Measure	Quantity	Weight	Calories	Day 1 Q C	Day 2 Q C	Day 3 Q C	Day 4 Q C	Day 5 Q C	Day 6 Q C	Day 7 Q C	Day 8 Q C	Day 9 Q C	Day 10 Q C
Soy Sauce Asparagus - Cooked	Cup	1		45	9	9	5	-	4 / 1 45	½ 25				
Hot Tea - Saccharin Green Beans, Cooked & Drained	Cup	1		30	4	4	4	4	4	4 / ½ 7				
Beets, Canned or Cooked, Peeled	Cup	1		85			1 85			1 85				
Broccoli, Cooked, Drained	Cup	1		40						½	1 40			
Brussells Sprouts, Cooked	Cup	1		55										
Cabbage, Celery, Onion Cabbage, Raw, Shredded	*Cup* Cup	*1* 1		*45* 15	(2) 113	(3) 135	1 45		1 45					
Cooked	Cup	1		30										
Carrots, Raw (5 1/2 x 1")	Ea	1		20			½ 10				1½ 5			
Cooked	Cup	1		45						¼ 10				
Cauliflower, Cooked, Buds	Cup	1		25							2 100			
Celery, Raw (8¼x1½" at root end)	Stk	1		5		3			3			*Sick*		
Corn, Sweet, Ear 5 x 1 3/4"	Ea	1		70				1 80						
Cucumbers, 7½"x2"	Ea	1		30			⅙ 5	⅙ 5	⅙ 5	5				
Lettuce, Iceberg, Raw 4-3/4"diam	Head	1		60			¼ 15	¼ 15	¼ 15	¼ 15	¼ 15			
Mushrooms, Canned or boiled	Cup	1		40	½ 20	½ 20	½ 20	½ 20	½ 20	½ 20				
Okra, Cooked, Pods 3x 5/8"	Pods	8		25										
Onions, *Green* Cooked	Cup	*1* 1		60			3							
Peppers, Sweet, Raw or Cooked	Ea	1		15							2			
Potatoes, Baked or Boiled, Peeled	Oz.	1		17	5½ 94 / 10 170	8 136 / 8 136	6½ 110 / 11 187	[illegible]	6 102 / 12 204	[illegible] 153 / 6 102	6 102 / [illegible]			
Radishes, Raw, Small	Ea	1		1							1			
Sauerkraut, Canned	Cup	1		45										
Spinach, Cooked *Soup*	Cup	1		45					15		1 50			
Squash, Summer, Cooked	Cup	1		30										
Tomatoes, Raw, Diam. 3", 2-1/8"hg / Cooked	ea / Cup	1 / 1		40 / 50	1 50	50	½ 50 / 1 30	1 30	¼ 15	1 25	1 25			
Total Calories Per Day					460	493	519	638	477	451	479	-0-		165
Weight Loss Per Day					171 0	171 0	168 3	168 0	167 1	167 0	166 1		165 1	6

CHAPTER V

GLUTTONY

In many of our crusades there is a time when we ask those who are still smoking if they would like to be delivered by the power of God, and there is a great response. At a meeting in Vallejo, California, an alcoholic was fantastically delivered by the power of God. At the next meeting a lady came up to me and said, "Why is it that you always pray for people to be delivered of cigarettes, you pray for them to be delivered of alcohol, but you never pray for the fat people!" God really spoke to me and I said, "All right, Lord, if that's what you want me to talk about this morning, that's what I'll talk about."

I have prayed for a lot of fat people, but this was the first time I had ever spoken on this subject at a meeting. I remembered that somewhere in Proverbs in the King James version there was a very interesting verse about fat. I think it's the one we all know and most of us ignore, because it really hits the foodaholic right between the eyes. I know why I didn't like it and why I didn't ever refer to it! It absolutely was a thorn in my flesh. I didn't know exactly where the verse was. I knew it was somewhere in Proverbs, and I also knew it was in King James. I said to the pastor, "Would you loan me your King James?" because I didn't have one with me that day. As he handed it to me it opened to the 23rd chapter of Proverbs. The first verse nearly floored me, even though it wasn't the one I was looking for, because this is exactly what it said: "When thou sittest to eat with a ruler (who is the ruler of this world? Satan is, of course), consider diligently what is before thee:" All I could see was a banquet table filled with mashed potatoes, gravy, corn on the cob loaded with butter, lasagna, spaghetti, salad with Rocquefort dressing on it, hot rolls with butter dripping all over them, pecan pie with whipped cream, bowls of nuts and mints and candies sitting around all over the place. "Consider diligently what is before thee;" That's all I could see. I said, "Well, Lord, I never knew that this was in the Bible. Tell me some more."

I read the next verse, and I couldn't believe what I read. It said, "and put a knife to thy throat, if thou be a man given to appetite." I said, "Now Lord, I know you don't intend for us to slit our throats just because we eat too much." Then, God said to me exactly what he meant. He said, "That's exactly what you're doing when you overeat! You are just cutting your own throat and cutting years off your life." (Read what the actuarial charts say about this same subject.) I read verse 3. It said, "Be not desirous of his dainties: for they are deceitful meat."

How many times have we eaten these super-elegant foods we know are fattening and have kidded ourselves into thinking, "Today we eat, tomorrow we diet!" I couldn't believe what I was reading here: "Be not desirous of his dainties; for they are deceitful meat." Isn't it amazing that those little dainties can tell us they are not going to hurt us? Isn't it amazing how convincingly those little dainties can tell us they are not going to stick on our bodies all the rest of our lives?

I love what Graham Kerr says: "You can eat a hot fudge sundae with whipped cream and nuts on it on any diet." I said, "You can?" He said, "Yes, if you only eat ONE bite." Not one bite after another and another and another, but just one bite each meal.

I have another real interesting saying: "It looks better on the plate than it does on me." I saw it on me for too many years, and I didn't really like what I saw. So, "be not desirous of his dainties: for they are deceitful meat." Don't let them lie to you. Who is the biggest liar of all? Satan, the ruler of this earth! In him there is no truth.

The next time you sit down at your table, consider diligently what is before thee. Look at each item before you and say, "Jesus, how little can I get by with, not how much can I eat?" Ask God to loose you from that appetite because he has a lot more to say in that same little chapter. I read the whole chapter, and by the time I got down to verse 20 I found what I thought I was looking for; and yet I felt that I had found something much better in the very beginning part. Verse 20 says, "Be not among winebibbers; among riotous eaters of flesh:" (The Revised Standard Version used "meat" instead of "flesh.") I think of what a riotous eater of flesh I was for many years. I loved to eat, and had a riotous time doing it!

Look at what verse 21 says is going to happen to you. It says, "for the drunkard and the glutton," and GOD PUTS THE ALCOHOLIC AND THE FOODAHOLIC IN EXACTLY THE SAME CATEGORY, "shall come to poverty: and drowsiness shall clothe a man with rags." Who doesn't get sleepy when he eats too much? Did you ever think back about some of the Thanksgiving dinners you've had? The table has been so loaded down it absolutely creaked, and you ate so much the only thing you could do was to get up and lie down and take a nap. That's what we used to do after every Thanksgiving dinner — see how much we could eat and then everybody had to take a nap. We were absolutely exhausted and overcome with drowsiness, just because we ate too much. Isn't it interesting that we look down upon the alcoholic, and yet God puts the glutton in exactly the same category.

Well, maybe you're like I am. Maybe you still keep telling little fibs and keep saying to yourself, "I'm really not a glutton." (I said that for years.) I used to think of a glutton as someone like King Henry VIII who tackled a whole leg of lamb with both hands and an open mouth, but never realized it could be someone like me who had better manners and tackled it with a knife and fork!

I think one of the most exciting things that ever happened to me in my whole life was when I finally admitted that I was a glutton. I like to eat, I like a tremendous amount of food, and I like all good rich, gooey stuff that you have no business eating! Therefore, I am a foodaholic. If I am a foodaholic, then I have been a glutton all my life, because I have eaten far more than I ever should have.

Thank you Jesus, because you made me honest. Ask God to tell you right now if you are a glutton. Ask God to turn his searchlight on the inside of you so that you can honestly see yourself and the amount of food you eat. YOU CAN NEVER GET HONEST WITH GOD UNTIL YOU ARE HONEST WITH YOURSELF. Are you really willing to admit the truth and say, "Lord, I'm a mess. I can't do it. I have tried it all these years, and I have miserably failed, because I am a foodaholic." I believe your first step for deliverance will come just exactly the way it came to me, when I was honest and admitted being a foodaholic. I believe there is only one answer for the alcoholic, and that's Jesus. The same Jesus who can deliver an alcoholic, who can deliver a dope addict, can deliver a food addict just as well. If you're one of them, would you like to pray a prayer with me right now?

"Lord Jesus, I am a foodaholic. I recognize that my problem is overeating and not a glandular problem. I admit that I like food. I admit that I love all kinds of rich food. I admit that I love too much of the kinds of food that puts weight on me. I have tried diets, Lord Jesus, and they haven't worked, because I've been doing them on my own with my carnal self, still desiring the things that I wasn't eating; but this time, Lord Jesus, I give you my appetite. I give you my desires, and I ask you to give me YOUR desires so that I will not overeat. Lord Jesus, help me to eat what I need to eat, but help me to see how little I can get by with, not how much can I eat. Lord Jesus, I'm going to thank you right now for retraining my eating habits so that I can get my weight down to where it should be.''

CHAPTER VI

WHERE DO WE GO FROM HERE?

If you sincerely prayed that prayer, there is the same wonder now that came into your heart when you asked Jesus to come in and be your Savior and Lord . . . "Where do we go from here?" This is where I think we really need some teaching and some understanding to know where we really are going to go from here. If two people with exactly the same strength were having a battle, it would end up to be a draw, wouldn't it? If they both have the same strength, they both have the same intelligence, they both have the same abilities, it would end up "no contest." Remember, however, ". . . greater is he that is in you, than he that is in the world." (I John 4:4 KJV) So, we know that we have the power of God within us to make us an overcomer.

This means an overcomer of all things, not just some things, but *all* things. That includes our appetites as well. You see, when the carnal self tries to overcome the carnal desires, we meet defeat; but Jesus gives us spiritual desires which can defeat the carnal desires. You can never have victory when you let your carnal desire and your carnal nature have the upper hand. You can *never* win the battle as long as you are trying to let your carnal nature diet for you. I believe this is the reason so many diets fail, because we try to do them in the flesh. This is impossible, because your carnal nature is there to tell you, "Just a little bit more won't hurt. Go ahead and eat it." That's your carnal nature in there that's always going to be battling what you're trying to do on your own.

Let's see what God has to say in Romans about this. Let's look in the Living Bible again at chapter 7, starting with verse 21:

> ROMANS 7
>
> [21] It seems to be a fact of life that when I want to do what is right, I inevitably do what is wrong. [22] I love to do God's will so far as my new nature is concerned; [23] [24] [25] but there is something else deep within me, in my lower nature, that is at war with my mind and wins the fight and makes me a slave to the sin that is still within me. In my mind I want to be God's willing servant but instead I find myself still enslaved to sin.
>
> So you see how it is: my new life tells me to do right, but the old nature that is still inside me loves to sin. Oh, what a terrible predicament I'm in! Who will free me from my slavery to this deadly lower nature? Thank God! It has been done by Jesus Christ our Lord. He has set me free.

Praise God! Jesus is the one who has set you free. Aren't you glad you prayed that prayer?

CHAPTER VII

THE DEVIL IS A SWEET LIAR

Proverbs 9:17, "Stolen waters are sweet, and bread eaten in secret is pleasant." (KJV)

Probably the first fifty times I read this in Proverbs, I couldn't understand why God would say, "Stolen waters are sweet, and bread eaten in secret is pleasant." That's not what God said at all. God merely indicated that this is what the prostitute was saying to the simpleton as he walked down the street. God never said that stolen waters were sweet. It was a prostitute speaking, who was, of course, lying, because the devil is a liar; and in him there is no truth.

One of the funniest things in the world, I think, is why many fat people stand in the kitchen and eat that extra peach or piece of candy, a bag of chips, or a cookie, and think, "Well, this isn't going to count, because I didn't eat it at a meal. It isn't going to count, because nobody sees me eating it, and it's only a little snack, anyway." The funny thing is, your body knows you ate it, and God sees you eating it. The way he has set up our metabolism or whatever it is that controls our weight, a calorie is still a calorie is still a calorie! Regardless of how you sneak it or how secretly you eat it or whatever time of the day or night you eat it, it is still a calorie.

I think of the food I have eaten over the sink. I don't really mean that I sat down and ate at the sink, but what about the goodies I snacked on as I was preparing a meal? Even though I am not a nibbler of the actual food that I cook, I was a great eater of other things. I think of how many times as I wrapped the sweet rolls for the freezer (for Charles) that I ate two in the process, or if I was really hungry, even three. Now, why should a mind that is supposed to be fairly intelligent (although I do doubt it at times) have a thought that said "Nobody saw you eat it, so you won't gain weight." Isn't the devil a BIG liar! And so was I . . . I was playing hide-and-seek with myself and God, hiding my secret snacks, and seeking his help to lose weight at the same time!

You know, one of the biggest downfalls of every person is believing that the devil is not a sweetie! This isn't true at all. The number of calories that are in a piece of cake, pie or candy are absolutely unbelievable. How many of you have snacked on a candy bar thinking "I was so hungry I had to have something." Do you realize that when you put that candy bar in your mouth, what you did was eat more calories than you should have eaten at your entire dinner? It was just something to "tide" you over until you ate. I know because I've eaten two, three and even four candy bars before a meal. You have to remember that I am a foodaholic. Maybe you only ate one, but I could eat up to five. As a matter of fact, I could finish a complete meal and turn right around and eat another meal without ever even batting an eyelash. This may sound impossible, but it's not. It's ridiculous, but not impossible.

I've tried eating the candies that you're supposed to eat before a meal, because they curb your appetite. I could eat a whole box, and it never curbed mine! I could go right on eating everything else that I had planned for dinner. In many of us there is a tremendous desire for sweets. Maybe mine dates back to that little girl looking in the ice cream parlor, just wishing that I could have all those little goodies that were in there. Maybe it was because I didn't have enough of these things when I was little. I don't really know. It doesn't make any difference. The question is, "What am I going to do about it TODAY, RIGHT NOW, when I can't afford to eat all those sweet things?"

You see, the devil really is a "false" sweetie. He can disguise himself as a candy bar. He can be a piece of fudge loaded with nuts. He can be a cake, with gooey frosting on it. He can be a pudding. He can be a Bavarian cream. He can be a pecan pie. The devil can be any of those kind of things, but I really believe if we turn our eyes upon Jesus and say, "the longer I serve him, the sweeter he grows," the less problem we'll have believing that the devil is a false sweetie and a bitter liar. Sweets are used by the devil, because they put on weight, although God doesn't intend for us to do without these delicacies. He expects us to eat them IN MODERATION! (That's a word that a foodaholic doesn't know!)

Look back at that little verse of scripture, and see what it says. "Stolen waters are sweet." Do you know what I think about stolen waters in this instance where it refers to a fat person? It's that candy bar that you sneaked when nobody was looking so that no one would know you had eaten it. It was an extra dessert you ate before you put dessert on the table for everybody else. It was the extra cup of pudding you put to one side to save for yourself when nobody else was looking. It's that candy store you went in and bought just a couple of pieces of candy because you were getting tired and you needed something to restore your energy. It's that ice cream you eat at midnight before you go to bed.

Look at the rest of this verse. It says, "bread eaten in secret is pleasant." That's why the foodaholic enjoys those secret snacks! They're eaten in secret! But that's the devil talking! Did you ever notice that when someone doesn't want anybody to know about something, they do it alone? Did it ever dawn on you when a person is going to have an affair outside of marriage it is always done at night when no one is looking, always done secretly (until they get caught). I've never seen or heard of a couple who were having a clandestine affair who got up in the middle of Main Street and announced to the whole world they were having an illicit love affair. They sneak around, under the cover of darkness, thinking that no one is going to see them; and therefore they'll get by with it. That's why we think that bread eaten in secret is so pleasant. (Or a drink enjoyed alone is fabulous!)

I imagine if we looked psychologically at a criminal we'd see he gets a real fiendish delight when he thinks he gets by with something. When he robs a bank and nobody catches him and nobody sees him, he takes tremendous pride in himself. Did you ever notice most crime is committed at night? Remember it's the devil, not God, who says "bread eaten in secret is pleasant." The same thing applies to all of those little goodies that we eat in secret, that we don't tell anyone about. However, we reap what we sow, as we wonder why we continue to gain weight.

Right now I'm laughing because I just thought "I wonder how many calories I would have logged up if I had put down all the extra little goodies I ate before it was actually meal time." I think of all the bags of taco-flavored chips I have eaten on the way home from the grocery store, just because I love them. I think of all the bags of corn chips I've eaten. I think of the bananas I've eaten in the car on the way home from the store. I think of a lot of other little goodies that I have eaten, not because I needed them, but just because I had to have something to "tide" me over until mealtime. I acted as if Jesus weren't enough.

So the devil really is a counterfeit sweetie. Who wants the devil for a sweetheart? I don't. Do you? I want Jesus all the way.

The devil tries to tell us if we eat a little something sweet it will satisfy us. Did you ever notice when you are on a hunger binge and the hunger pangs are really gnawing at your stomach, the thing that you THINK satisfies you the most is something sweet. We run to the refrigerator and look for that extra piece of pie left over from last night, or we look in the cupboard for that candy bar. Do you know that your taste buds respond to sweetness faster than anything else? This is why we think that something sweet is going to satisfy us. Do you also know that the taste disappears from your sweet buds faster than it does from anything else? We have four different senses of taste — sour, bitter, sweet and salt. The sweet bud is the one that responds the quickest and disappears the fastest. How about that?

The next time you are tempted to take something sweet, Graham Kerr recommends you try a bite of salami with an olive wrapped on the inside, because that will satisfy your taste buds for the next three hours. Just as sin enjoyed for a fleeting moment is followed by guilt, so is a bite of sweets which only lasts moments followed by pounds which linger long after!

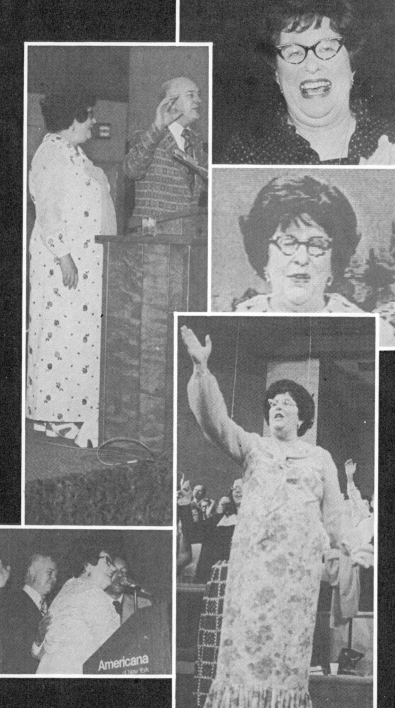

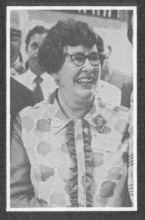

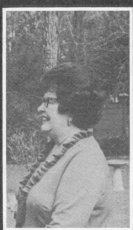

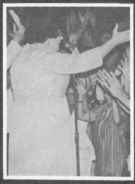

BEFORE

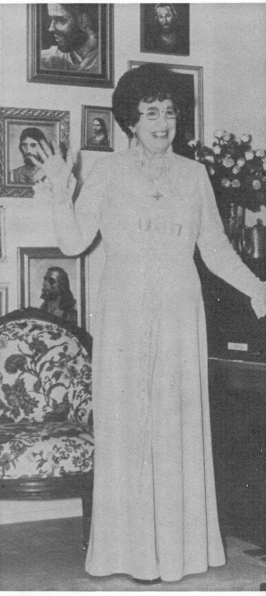

AFTER

THANK YOU JESUS! HALLELUJAH! Frances praising God in front of the "Jesus" wall in their home.

CHAPTER VIII

THE GREAT SUBSTITUTION

When I became a Christian, I substituted Jesus for sin! II Corinthians 5:21 says, "For he (God) hath made him (Christ) to be sin for us, who knew no sin; that we might be made the righteousness of God in him." I especially like this in the Living Bible, because I can just visualize two test tubes with Jesus and his perfection in one and me and my blackness in another. The Living Bible puts it so beautifully, because it says, "For God took the sinless Christ and poured into him our sins. Then, in *exchange*, he poured God's goodness into us!"

Wasn't that really a fantastic exchange? You exchange one thing for another, or you substitute. In other words, I substituted Jesus Christ for sin. I exchanged my sins for God's goodness, according to the word of God. I exchanged (or substituted) a lot of "my" things for the things of God. I traded my cigarettes for the privilege of loving Jesus more. I substituted God's new wine for the martinis that I used to drink.

The same thing applies to every area of our life. I want you to look at food. There is a very exciting way we can substitute good food for fat! You may be just like I am. I prayed and prayed and prayed for years for God to take weight off of me or to keep me from gaining weight. Yet, there is that physical part, that human part, that is involved when God tells us to do certain things. Because of this, I learned to play a substitution game where food is concerned. And just as I learned in life that the substitution was far better than the original (Jesus and me), so in food the same thing holds true. You might want to learn how, too!

I sincerely recommend with all my heart that you learn some of the nutritive values of food from the USDA chart reproduced in part in the back of this book. Charles and I have learned to make an exciting game out of substituting. I might be thinking about pork chops, so I immediately look at the calorie counter and discover that pork chops have an almost unbelievable amount of calories. This is when we begin to play the substitution game. I think "What else would I like to have just as well, but which has 1/3 the calories?" It doesn't take me very long when I look at the calorie chart to discover that I can have something just as good, and just as satisfying, but which does not have the calories that the pork chop does. We have baked chicken and mushrooms instead!

You'll discover it gets to be a real challenge to find the foods you can substitute and still please your family. I've discovered some of the best vegetables in the world are the ones that have the least calories. I've also discovered that you can do a tremendous amount for the low-calorie vegetables and make them taste different each time. A diet for God is one of the most exciting challenges in the world. I want to really encourage you to accept the challenge right now!

Make food substitution a fascinating game! If you feel an urge for candied sweet potatoes, the best way I know of to get rid of the urge is to discover that one small candied sweet potato has 295 calories! The same amount of turnips has only 35. Lord, give me the turnips, and make me love them just as much! At first glance, the sweet potato is a real enemy, but if you look further, you'll find it chuck full of vitamins. Don't banish it forever, but lay it to one side temporarily, since your immediate goal is weight loss, but what God wants for you is complete health.

While we're on the subject of substitutions, I know there are times, especially when you're starting on a food retraining program (that's a better name than dieting) you'll really get hungry and think you're going to starve if you don't have something to eat. I formerly felt the best thing to eat was a raw carrot or a piece of celery. I discovered that this didn't satisfy the hunger pang I had. It didn't do a thing for me! I'm going to suggest that you think about substituting a small amount of protein for that carrot.

Definitely stay away from sweets! Definitely stay away from bread! The only thing you'll have to do is really pray for the first few minutes, because it takes a few minutes for the protein to get into your system and make you realize that you've really had something to eat. Hang in there, because the real problem can come from the overeating you do by being impatient and not waiting for nature to let your brain know that your stomach has had something put into it. Also remember this, if you start nibbling in sin, soon you will be eating, then overeating, THEN FAT! Did you ever notice that you got hungrier after you nibbled? YES, YOU GET HUNGRIER WHEN YOU NIBBLE!

A good idea is to keep cold broiled chicken breasts in your refrigerator. I love them! If you're hungry, you can reach in for a 1 oz. bite, and that's only 37½ calories. You'd be surprised how much chicken there is in one ounce. It's surprising how a little bit of this can really tide you over until you sit down to eat whatever your meal is at night. Retrain your appetite as quickly as possible to wean yourself from snacks. REMEMBER, NIBBLING MAKES YOU HUNGRIER!!

One morning as Charles and I were eating breakfast

and he was eating a lot of goodies while I was still on the Daniel fast, I said "Do you realize that yours looks so much better than mine, tastes so much better than mine, is so much more fattening than mine, and yet in ten minutes our stomachs will both feel exactly the same? Mine will probably even feel better than yours!" Remember that when you're tempted to cheat. Just hang in there for 10 minutes, and you'll never know the difference!

Back to snacks, I made Charles a guacamole salad one day while we were home because it's one of his favorite dishes. (A real no-no for dieters). I gave him a sample on a corn chip and he said it was super delicious. About noon he got up from his desk for something and his mind recalled how good the guacamole was and his thoughts went to the refrigerator. Because we have never gone back to the bondage of 3 meals a day since we went on the Daniel fast, his stomach really didn't reflect hunger, and he had no reason to eat, nor did he have a desire. His mind had sent a recalled signal to his taste buds and they convinced his MIND that he should have a few bites. He wasn't dieting, so he ate more than a few bites because it was so good. He commented while he was eating it that, like in sports, he was breaking training — "skipping lunch training."

At about the same time the next day, sure enough his stomach had hunger desires. It's so easy to retrain our eating habits and be happy, but when we break training, we interfere with the timing mechanism of our brain and the contentment we had is interrupted with a lust for unnecessary food consumption. This is the time to have a cup of hot tea. Snacks flirt with your taste buds, leading them into temptation.

I went on a frankfurter diet once — maybe you've been on the same thing! Didn't lose any weight, but sure had fun eating hot dogs. But do you know what a shocking discovery I made about one of America's favorites?

THEY'RE JUST LOADED WITH CALORIES!!! The regular small frankfurter (8 per pound) has 170 calories in it. Would you believe that? Add the bun to it and you've got another 120 calories, or a total of 290 without adding catsup, onions, etc. And chili . . . well, that puts you completely out of the ballpark, because 1/2 cup is 255 calories. Who would ever suspect a chili dog contained so much caloric sin! It's amazing how fast you can learn to substitute when you discover the truth about certain foods.

Lamb chops are on a lot of diets, but I discovered that one chop, weighing 4.8 ounces has 400 calories. That's a lot of calories to put in your body at one time with one little piece of meat. And remember part of that is bone, too. There are lots of meats you can substitute that will be delicious. Try 4 ounces of boneless ham for only 246 calories.

Start looking for the food that gives you the most satisfaction for the weight! It's amazing to me how little a shrimp weighs. I discovered that you can eat 26 to 28 medium shrimp, 3 to 3½ ounces, and have something like 140 calories. Watch not only the weight of what you eat, but watch the quantity that you actually get, because some foods weigh heavier than others. As I mentioned earlier, chicken is another food that weighs "light."

Everyone ought to know the truth about some of the foods that are the real killers. Would you believe that one piece of pecan pie has 490 calories (and that's without whipping cream). Would you believe that one little wedge of cheese cake without topping also has 495 calories. Would you believe that one little piece of mincemeat pie has 365 calories? Probably the best kind of pie to indulge in, if you feel you must indulge, is pineapple chiffon. One piece of that has only 265 calories. The exciting thing about this food retraining program, however, is that you can have dessert! YOU CAN HAVE ANY KIND OF DESSERT

YOU WANT! One bite! No more . . . just one bite! You'll soon discover how that one little bite will completely satisfy you if you start by saying "One bite is all I'm going to eat."

Charles and I eat in cafeterias whenever possible because it's easy to watch your calories there. He always lets me pick the dessert and I pick the most scrumptious one available. After I've eaten my dinner, he gives me the first bite of the dessert, and he eats the rest! I'm perfectly satisfied because of the food retraining program in my body. Thank you Jesus!

Pancakes are another calorie surprise, because one pancake has only sixty calories, but do you know what the problem is? It isn't the pancake that's fattening. It's the syrup and the butter and goo that you put on it. An actual pancake itself, if you like to eat them plain, is just sixty calories, that's all. Try them with salt and pepper sometime — you might be surprised. Charles loves them with bacon and eggs, and they appetizingly hold longer than bread.

And talking about bread, look at what it does to you! One cloverleaf roll has 120 calories. A commercial pan roll has 85 calories, and the bun you put a hamburger on adds 120 calories. One hard roll has 155 calories. Two little whole-grain rye wafers, 1⅞" x 3½" have 45 calories.

Do you know where the real dillies are? In the fat and oil department. Did you know that one beautiful little stick of butter contains 810 calories? Multiply that times four in a pound and you have 3,240 calories! No wonder we get fat in a land of plenty where we smear butter on everything, and we season everything with butter. Maybe you're one of those people who, like I, thought that margarine had a lot less calories than butter. It might be cheaper, but it's not any cheaper in calories. As a matter of fact, it's more, because each stick of margarine contains 815 calories, or five more than a stick of butter. A pound has 3,260. Don't be fooled into thinking that just because you eat margarine it's not nearly as fattening.

I want you to take a peek at cooking oils, regardless of what kind you use. Corn oil, cotton seed oil, olive oil, peanut oil, safflower oil or soy bean oil, all have the same caloric content. In each cup there are 1,945 calories. No wonder we get so fat when we eat french fried potatoes, french fried fish and french fried onion rings. Remember a calorie is a calorie is a calorie, no matter how you try to cover it up and ignore the fact that you cooked it in oil, even if you tried to drain the excess off the french fries.

One of the best substitutes I know is to substitute some kind of fruit for whatever sweet you think you've got to have. You can eat a beautiful half of a grapefruit and have only 45 calories as against 490 for the pecan pie. Be careful that you don't get carried away and buy canned fruit, because most of them have a syrup pack, which brings the content for one cup up to 180 calories. Lord, let me look for the water pack or try always to get the fresh fruit! (And the same thing applies to vegetables — always use fresh whenever possible!)

One of the foods that really sustained me on my personal food retraining program has been apples. The average size apple (3 per pound) contains only 70 calories which is a beautiful dessert. I cut the apple into tiny little slivers and squeeze the juice of a lemon on them. When you cut a whole apple into little wedges, it looks like you have a BIG dessert, and the lemon juice brings out the flavor of the apples. Be sure to leave the skin on because the effort you use to chew the skin helps get rid of some of the calories. You can eat two apples a day for 140 calories, or have dessert twice a day, for less than 1/3 of a piece of cheese cake. Hallelujah!

Bananas are a little more fattening, but they're not as bad as you think. One medium banana has 100 calories. Cantalope is an excellent calorie friend because a half has only 60 calories. Would you believe, though, that cranberry sauce, that good accompaniment to our Thanksgiving and Christmas meals, has 405 calories in one single little cup?

Let's look away from that and look at something that can be just as good but not have as many calories. You can have three apricots — this is about 1/4 pound, for only 55 calories. Be careful of the dried, uncooked fruit because they're really loaded. One cup of those is 390 calories. Also watch out for those that are canned in heavy syrup!

Fresh pineapple is a calorie bargain. One cup of the raw, diced pineapple is only 75 calories. If you buy the syrup pack pineapple, watch out! One cup of crushed pineapple has 195 calories, 2 small or 1 large slice, 90. Four prunes have 70 calories. A half-ounce package of raisins has 40 calories. Raw raspberries are real good, because one cup has only 70 calories. Strawberries are another real blessing, because one cup has 90 calories. They do an excellent job of satisfying your urge for something sweet.

One cup of brown sugar has 820 calories! White sugar, 770. Think twice before you use it. Mayonnaise has 100 for each tablespoon you use (and this doesn't mean heaped up). Substitute a low calorie dressing. The one I use has only 16. Quite a difference, isn't it? The french dressing I use has only 2 per tablespoon. The regular kind has 65. Watch out, though, because all dressings labeled "low calorie" are not necessarily extremely low.

Play the great substitution game in your house for every meal! And substitute Bible reading with a glass of skim milk for that noon meal. You can get along beautifully with spiritual food instead of physical food. By eliminating the noon meal in our house we figured we would have time to write 5 new books next year with just the time saved in the preparation of lunch, eating and cleaning up, to say nothing of the shopping time saved! Hallelujah! Reading the Bible can be far more nourishing without putting on weight.

This can be the most exciting venture you've ever undertaken in your life. GOD CAN HEAL YOUR APPETITE! He controls the universe and he's bigger than your appetite. Remember it's your appetite which needs reducing — the fat body will fall in line. We have not let the food retraining program in our house become a drudge. It has been FUN all the way because we were doing it for Jesus! I've had a lot of interesting conversations with him, especially in the beginning because I'd say "Jesus, is this ALL I get to eat?" And he'd smile back and say, "My grace is sufficient for your needs." And I'd be content. He'll do the same for you. There is joy in the Lord, even when you're retraining your eating habits. We had fun the other day in a restaurant ordering one small steak and two plates. It was advertised as an 8 ounce steak, and each of us only needed 4 ounces, so look at the economic saving we made there. If we'd all conserve on our food budget, think what it could do for a hungry world!

Charles even said he loves the "lesser me" more because I'm much healthier and happier and have more energy to love him than I ever had before . . . another Hallelujah for the great substitution!

Think about this:

Sabbath was made for man, not man for the sabbath!
Food was made for man, not man for food!
Eat to live, not live to eat!
"JESUS, HOW MUCH CAN I LOVE THE RETRAINING PROGRAM, NOT HOW MUCH DO I SUFFER!"

Train your attitudes — Think GOOD, not BAD! Pray each time you seek knowledge, and be sure and thank God for each substitution discovery.

CHAPTER IX
LEARN THE LAW!

The sixth chapter of Romans really spoke to me concerning dieting. I want you to start with the twelfth verse. It says, "Do not let sin (appetite) control your puny body any longer; do not give in to its sinful desires."

Drop down to verse 16. "Don't you realize that you can choose your own master? You can choose sin *(food)*(with death)*(fat)* or else obedience (with acquittal)*(or obedience with a weight loss)*. The one to whom you offer yourself — he will take you and be your master, and you will be his slave."

Paul had quite a bit to say about the law, and it's interesting he felt the law was really a good thing. Turn to the 7th chapter of Romans, verse 7, and see what it says. "Well then, am I suggesting that these laws of God are evil? Of course not!" We all know that one of the laws of God is that if you overeat, you're going to gain weight. Look what it says, "No, the law is not sinful but it was the law that showed me my sin." You see, the one who really convicted me was the Holy Spirit, but his convicting power became strong when I learned the law on food and discovered how outright sinful certain foods are! I think the day I discovered the number of calories chili had was the last time I ate chili. Just think, one little cup without beans is 510 calories. One cup of chili is about half of a bowl. So in a bowl of chili you get about 1,000 calories. (And that doesn't count the crackers . . . 12½ calories EACH.) Help, Lord! And thank you for making me lose my appetite for chili.

You have no idea how much better fish looked after I discovered the caloric catastrophe in chili! Canned salmon (3 oz.) has only 120 calories. Isn't that a lot better than 1,000? Look at shrimp — 3 oz., 100 calories. You can eat TEN CANS OF SHRIMP or 30 ounces of shrimp for the same number of calories that one bowl of chili contains. Look how much more shrimp will do for your waistline. And at the same time you're thinking about that, think of the heartburn you won't have. One of the greatest number of requests for prayer are by people who are overweight and request me to pray for their heartburn and gas problems. Hallelujah, learn the law and you'll dispense with these problems.

Please remember I am not a dietician. I am not a doctor. I only know what happened in my own life. I cannot tell you what to do, but I can let you know what worked in my life. I learned a very interesting lesson about the law this morning. If you lose weight, you're going to need a smaller size in your dresses. I took a dress to the dressmaker this morning that was made ten months ago, and discovered that ten whole beautiful inches had to be cut out from both the waist and hips. Praise Jesus! Was learning the law worth while? It certainly was!

Rib roast, when served 1/4" thick, weighs about 1/2 pound per serving. Calories — 1,000 or more! What does the law tell you to do with that? Ignore it for chicken or fish. Charles loves it, so he had one recently and gave me a small piece right out of the center. Delicious, but that was all I wanted!

I want you to check on the so-called dieter's specials. This usually consists of four ounces of hamburger (supposedly lean) and one half cup of cottage cheese with one peach on a lettuce leaf. I have been fooled into thinking this was really one of the extremely low calorie dinners. Now watch: 4 ounces of hamburger has 245 calories. One half cup cottage cheese, 180. One half peach (syrup packed is what they usually give in a restaurant), 100 calories, making a grand total of 525 calories. This is before you have anything to drink.

The more I discover the caloric content in foods, the more the "law" convicts me and the more I change my eating habits. That's why I hope you'll refer to the "law" (caloric chart) in the back of this book every time you sit down to prepare a meal or think about food.

Another tremendous verse of scripture is Matthew 26:41 (KJV) "Watch and pray, that ye enter not into temptation: the spirit indeed is willing, but the flesh is weak." Think how true this is. How many times do we pass by a store that has some real super goodies in it, and we discover that we have fallen into temptation, because we are irresistibly drawn in to buy some of whatever that little goodie is in there. I know, because for a long time I had a "thing" about the airport in Chicago. In my opinion they have the best Polish hot dogs anywhere in the USA. We always looked forward to eating one whenever we had to make a change of planes in Chicago. We always found time to stop and run by the Polish hot dog counter and pick up one. I have no idea how many calories they have, but I just don't walk by there any more. I walk on the outside as far away as I can, and I haven't been the least bit tempted nor have I felt that I missed anything.

We really need to be careful of the things we actually look at, because all of the packaging that is done today, and all the cakes and pies that are pictured on packages are done to stimulate your taste buds, so that your saliva glands will really get into action. Did you ever notice if you go to the store hungry you are much more tempted to buy sinful things? I'd say, "REALLY watch and pray that you won't enter into temptation." Watch what time you go to the store. The best time is after your BIG breakfast!

You're going to have to watch what departments you go by, and I would really ignore going by that bakery department until you get all of the fat off that you want. I'd ignore the cookie department. It's no good for fat people, because if you're like me, I can't stop when I eat one cookie. I have to eat two, three, four or more. And even if you have to keep cookies in the house for your family, remember to listen to the Holy Spirit when he slaps your hands and says, "Get your hands out of that cookie jar." We all KNOW that the flesh is weak. That's why it's best to stay away from even looking at the things that are really wicked for the diet. "Resist the devil *(devil's food cake)*, and he will flee from you." Jas. 4:7 (KJV) Remember the motto is "JESUS, HOW LITTLE CAN I GET BY WITH, NOT HOW MUCH CAN I EAT!"

Another thing that creates a problems in many of us is, "What do we do when we go out to dinner?" May I tell you what we do? Traveling on the road as much as we do, we don't accept very many dinner invitations, because we give ourselves so completely to the Lord that there just isn't enough energy to go and eat at someone's home. Not only that, I have to be real honest and tell them that I am dieting. Anyone who loves you would not want you to undergo unnecessary hardships by watching others eat all kinds of delicious foods. In the early stages of your food retraining program you might discover it's best not to accept any dinner invitations, because every one of them will require tremendous "watching and praying," because it's so difficult to sit there and WATCH everyone else eat super-delicious things, while you sit there and nibble on a lettuce leaf and PRAY for your attitude! When your weight gets down to where it should be, you're going to be able to go out and eat with your friends IN MODERATION. But I really do believe that during that trying, testing period, which is when you are starting to lose weight and the devil is really testing you, the best thing to do is to flee from the devil as fast as you can. By that I mean stay away from even looking at things that are super-delightful, super-delicious and super-fattening. Watch and pray much.

If you really mean business with your goal for God, God will see to it that no temptation is ever so strong that he doesn't give you the power to overcome it. But the best way I know of is to stay away from even looking at all these super-good things or even going places where they are served. Look at what happened to me!

Charles and I had ministered at Rex Humbard's Cathedral of Tomorrow and when the meeting was over a group of us went to a delightful Jewish restaurant, specializing in whipped cream desserts. I was in a "coasting" period where dieting was concerned and discovered how weak the flesh can be! As we entered the front door there was a huge case of whipped cream delicacies! I made the fatal mistake of looking at them! The thing that really got my attention was a whipped cream puff. This was the biggest one I'd ever seen, and covered with the fudgiest frosting ever! My mouth watered! I asked the waitress if it was real whipped cream or just custard. She assured me it was thick whipped cream. I HAD TO HAVE ONE! I forgot that dieting is like Christianity — a 24 hour a day, 7 day a week thing!

Charles got a beautiful piece of cheese cake, and I got the whipped cream puff. I laughingly said "Lord, forgive me for the sin I'm about to eat." I ate half of Charles', and he ate half of mine. I enjoyed every single little bite because it was the most delicious sin I've ever eaten. Thick, sweet whipped cream on the inside, and fantastic fudge frosting on the outside. Never have I ever eaten anything that tasted as good as that whipped cream puff, and it was exactly what God wanted, because the minute I took the last bite, he said "Now how long are you going to have to diet to take that moment of delight off your stomach?" I almost got sick! In that moment of being tempted, I had to give up almost everything I should have eaten for the next two weeks. Was it worth it? No, it was not! Rex Humbard had said to me "I never order dessert, I let someone else do it, and then I take one bite." Next time, I'm going to have one bite of his. That's all. Hallelujah! Thank you Lord for teaching me a lesson I'll never forget!

Did you ever notice how people will try to break down every wall that you have built up against overeating? They'll say "Oh, honey, you're not too fat." Did anybody ever tell you that? People used to tell me that all the time. They would say, "Well, after all, Frances, you're a BIG woman. You carry your weight well. You're not overweight." Sometimes you can sort of salve your pride and think, "Well, that's right, I really am a BIG woman." In my case, I am. I think my bones alone would weigh more than the average woman will weigh in her lifetime, but that's one of the things I have to put up with. My mother and daddy had a big frame, therefore I have a big frame, too. There isn't any way I can get rid of the frame, but it's up to me how much I put on that big frame.

Another favorite saying of our friends is "Oh, come on, eat just this little bit. It won't hurt you. You'll hurt my feelings if you don't eat this beautiful dessert I made just for you." The dessert probably has 500 to 1000 calories in it! That means trouble! I wonder if that same person would look at you and say "Come on, go to bed with Mr. Jones. It won't hurt you just this one time." Would that same person put a gun in your hand and say, "Just go over there and shoot Mr. Smith. It won't make any difference this one time!!" Who says it won't make any difference? Even our best-meaning friends can put us in an unholy spot by saying "Oh, go ahead and eat just a little bit." Let's don't cause our brother (or sister) to stumble even if it's only "angel food" cake they're stumbling over!

If you are a hostess who's having a dinner and your guest comes in and says to you that she's dieting or he's dieting, love them to death, don't be a stumbling block in their diet. Give them that little piece of lettuce they want or whatever they ask for, and then be happy. Enjoy their Christian fellowship, and don't worry about how few calories they eat!

Would you ask the alcoholic to have one little drink, telling him it wouldn't hurt just this once? Would you insist the cigaretteholic take a cigarette after Jesus had delivered him? Remember the foodaholic deserves the same consideration.

CHAPTER X

WHY DON'T I "WANT" TO LOSE WEIGHT?

I recently made a survey and asked a number of people a series of questions, one of which was the title of this chapter. The answers were interesting and revealing. What makes us think there isn't any reason to diet, or that it's a hopeless situation? I asked a young girl who was tremendously overweight why she didn't want to diet and she said "Who are you dieting for?" She had been married a relatively short while and her marriage had obviously been a great disappointment, so she was saying "Why should I bother losing weight for my husband because our marriage isn't very good." I suggested that she diet for her husband and she said "Why diet for him?" This is a very sad situation when we are willing to let ourselves go completely to pot just because some situation in our life isn't right. Getting fat won't make it any better. Did you ever notice how many people will say "Look at all the hypocrites in church. That's why I don't go." What they're really saying is "I'm going to let a sinner send me to hell." That's exactly what the young girl was saying "I'm going to let my husband send me to my grave early, because I'm going to eat so much to make up for the failure of our marriage that I'll get fat and die young."

The desires of your heart will make it possible for you

to lose weight. You have to honestly make a decision with your own mind, heart, body and soul, that you *WANT* God to help you lose weight. All the diets in the world won't help you until you are somehow motivated to "WANT" to lose weight. The Houston Chronicle, Tuesday, October 28, 1975, said: "Forty per cent of Americans have or will have a weight problem, and MOTIVATION is the key to losing excess baggage, a specialist in weight loss believes . . . . " Are you aware of the fact that most people are not willing to sacrifice the little bit that it might take in the beginning to get the weight started in the downward pattern?

I had recently asked a lot of people to start on a "Daniel fast" with me for the very simple reason I wanted to actually see what would happen to a group if they stayed on a "Daniel fast" for ten days. I first thought to myself "There's no way I can do this, because we're going to start on a tour at the end of the sixth day; and it's not possible when you're away from home to be able to get the vegetables you need." God said, "Don't ask anybody else to do it unless you do it yourself." I probably thought "But God, the CIRCUMSTANCES are all wrong for a 'Daniel fast.' " God didn't let me go, so on it I went, and for the next ten days, under the most inconvenient circumstances in the world, God gave me the supernatural will power I needed. I cannot claim any credit for myself, but give all the glory to God, because I survived without cheating one solitary bite. This is extremely hard when you are not in a position to get the food you need, and doubly hard when you go out to dinner with the Galloping Gourmet and his wife on one of these ten days and they take you to a fabulous Italian restaurant where they serve at least eight courses with every meal. Yet we had the most beautiful Christian fellowship in the world, and I ate only the things which were on my "Daniel fast" and nothing else.

I called the office to see how other people were

reacting to the "Daniel fast." One of the couples I had asked to go on the "Daniel fast" gave me a very interesting answer: "Well, the circumstances haven't been right. So we haven't been able to start on it." All I could think was "It isn't the circumstances that have to be right. It's the DESIRES that have to be right. The circumstances are *never* right."

It is NEVER the right time to start on a diet, because you either have something in the refrigerator that's too good to throw away, or you're having company and you don't want to sit there and not eat with them, or some other excuse. So the CIRCUMSTANCES are never right. They'll never be right tomorrow either. They won't be right a year from now. Get your desires in line, then your circumstances will be right. Remember what it says in the Bible, ". . . now is the day of salvation." The Bible doesn't say that tomorrow is the day of salvation or next week is the day of salvation, or that the day of salvation will be when the circumstances are right. It says, "NOW is the day of salvation." So NOW is the day for you to start your beautiful fast or diet, reformation movement, food retraining program, whatever you want to call it, so you can be what God wants you to be.

Dr. William Howard Hay, in his interesting book "How to always BE WELL" says "As you drift idly in the rapids of Niagara Falls and reason that since you are still afloat the danger of the falls is not so great as painted, better begin to row upstream at once, before it is too late, for the longer you drift, the closer comes the time when struggle against the current will be too difficult, perhaps impossible, and you will be swept down to certain destruction."

Remember, before the start on your diet, pray and ask God to give you the right attitude. Look on this as a great adventure! Look on it as a great challenge to make some real "blah" foods into the most delicious, healthy, weight

losing, exciting adventure in the world. God can do it for
YOU, when YOU do it for Jesus!

Sin on this earth started in the Garden of Eden when
Eve ate the forbidden fruit. I want you to really think about
that. This was never really brought to my mind until one
afternoon in Ellendale, North Dakota. Two women were
sitting in our room discussing the "fat" problem. One said
"You know, all of the sin of this earth really started with
food." And that's exactly where it all started. With food!
And food is still sin in the lives of a lot of us because we're
eating what we've been told not to eat!

Here's a verse of scripture that really spoke to my
heart. Philippians 3:18 & 19 (KJV) "For many walk, of whom
I have told you often, and now tell you even weeping, that
they are the ENEMIES OF THE CROSS OF CHRIST: Whose
end is destruction, whose God is their belly, and whose
glory is in their shame, who mind earthly things."

Did you hear what that said? I did! It said to me that I
had been an enemy of the cross of Christ when I was
miserably overweight. I said "God, let me NEVER, NEVER,
NEVER be an enemy of the cross of Christ!" The hardest
thing in the world to admit is the part that says "whose
God is their belly," but in my own life I had to admit that
this was true because of being a foodaholic! For years I
have not been able to lose weight, because secretly my
god was my belly. Praise God he has set me free! He has
loosed me from being controlled by another god!
Hallelujah!

Here are the most commonly used excuses for not
losing weight per the survey:
1. "My biggest problem with my weight was that I was
   told to finish my meal before I could have dessert."
2. "Food was given as a reward for well doing, and so
   when I eat a lot I think I've done well."
3. "I think my biggest problem was created when our
   family discussed problems while we ate. When my

dad threw a fit, it was always while we were eating, so we would all get upset and disturbed and we would eat more and more and faster and faster. Now when I get upset or troubled, I have to fight eating everything in sight."

4. "The biggest thing was when I broke up with a guy I was going to marry. I had emotional problems and loneliness, so to suppress the hurt, I ate and ate. Then it began to be a habit, a habit I couldn't break."

5. "I'm a single guy, about 150 pounds overweight. The reason I am overweight is that I was lonely, not a little, but a lot. My father was in the military, and I was taught not to have close friends, so I substituted food for friends. I got so overweight I tried to lose weight, but it didn't work. I tried everything. Then I got to the place that I thought 'It doesn't matter the way I look. People will have to accept me the way I am.' I didn't care, but now God has changed my attitude. I know only God can do it, because I've tried everything else."

6. "I ate because I was lonely and had no friends. That was the only way I could get rid of my loneliness."

Here's another very interesting letter that was sent to me. It was simply entitled:

Reasons for Overweight — Loneliness

and it listed the following:

1. A couple works, and one leaves the other one out — no car — no friends.

2. Couple spends time together but never FOR each other. With each other, but not REALLY with each other.

3. Parents who work.

4. Parents who spend all their time together, leaving the children out.

5. Left out by friends.

6. Overimportance of food all throughout life
    (a) I had all the money I needed to buy expensive food, so I treated my friends and ate with them — too often, too much, too rich!
    (b) Bad teaching of what good food really is
    (c) Baby cries for bottle, and this is used to satisfy other needs. Very important at all ages, because food is a substitute for many reasons.
    (d) Reward
    (e) Fear of never having enough:
        (1) Where will the next meal come from?
        (2) People are starving. Will I starve some day, too?
        (3) Time schedule. Will I have time to eat later on. If not, I'd better eat now. What happens? I eat later on, too.
        (4) A picture of doom, the end times when there's not enough food to go around.
    (f) Used to supply other needs, a need of love and a need of attention.
    (g) A Christian's way of killing oneself as an out for problems or lack of attention.
    (h) Told not to leave things on plate. You get punished if you do.
    (i) At the movie everybody gets popcorn.
    (j) Three meals a day are forced on us as a standard "

Then at the very end I love what the letter said:

"Real reason — none."

Along with this letter was another little chart which simply said: "Reasons for not losing." There were ten given.

1. Too much to lose. It's too long of a road.
2. I have no one to lose with.
3. I have no real purpose. Will Jesus really think it's neat if I lose weight?
4. Who will appreciate it?

5. What good would it do?
6. I've been this way my whole life long. Why change now?
7. Who really cares?
8. I have an obsession for food.
9. It's there. Why not eat it?
10. Everything that God made is good, so why not enjoy it?

I'm not going to comment on the reasons for not losing weight, but I'm going to ask you to just simply apply those reasons to your own life. Do any of them belong to you? Did you hear the poignant cry for help that came through this letter? Maybe these following short statements will help you and help the person who sent me the note: Look at the same number for the question and the answer!

1. Lose the first five pounds and LOØSE that feeling of self-pity!
2. Find yourself a partner. There are plenty of fat people around who would love to have you as a "fat" partner for skinny foods.
3. What about you? The Bible says to love your neighbor as you love yourself, and how can you love yourself when you know you're too fat
4. How about you?
5. It will give you a new outlook on life.
6. Why not?
7. God does, because he knows you're unhappy.
8. Let Jesus be your obsession.
9. It looks better on the plate than it does on me.
10. The Bible says, "All things in moderation."

We tell our children to eat everything that's on their plate because it's sinful or it's a waste to throw it away. How many times have we said "Don't waste that food. That food costs money. Don't waste that food! Daddy worked hard to make enough money to buy it. DON'T WASTE IT.

GOD'S ANSWER TO FAT . . . LOØSE IT!

We can't afford to waste things around this house because we're poor. Think of the hungry, starving people."

We recently had the opportunity to talk with the wife of the president of a college who had acquired a weight problem. She said God had just dealt with her about eating half of what was on her plate. She said she was really having difficulty, having been brought up in depression times to think it was really a sin to throw food down the sink or into the garbage disposal, but she herself decided it was far more of a sin to put weight on herself than it was to let food go down the drain! The moral of that story is "Don't put too much on your plate." And we really ought to start at the core. STOP COOKING TOO MUCH!

The real economy starts with what you buy and then how much of it you prepare. The amount of food that's thrown in the American garbage can is unbelievable. The food that's thrown in your garbage can, I'm sure is unbelievable. It's amazing what we could do if we would just stop to watch and "think before we cook," and "look (at calories) before we eat!" If you have plenty of money to buy too much food, buy less and eat less to make funds and food available to give to the hungry people of the world. One person can only do a little, but 200,000 can do a lot!

Ask God to really give you the desire because until you yourself make the decision and MEAN IT, there's nothing anyone can say to help you. It's hard for me to understand what turned the switch for me, until I began to realize the problem was not my weight, but my APPETITE which I hadn't been willing to give to God. When I sincerely gave THAT to him, he and he alone, took away the desire for food, and he'll do it for you too!

CHAPTER XI
THE WRAP UP

Quit blaming everyone else for your problem! Admit that the fault lies with you. Quit blaming your parents for the fact that you are short and stocky. You might inherit your height from your parents, but what you hang on that height depends on you. You've probably always been overweight because of a family habit of eating too much. The time to break that habit is RIGHT NOW! And the person to break that habit is YOU! I know it's hard, because I've suffered all the pangs of hunger that you have. For 5 years I said to Charles "Honey, you don't understand what it's like to be hungry all the time." The hunger really wasn't in my stomach, it was in my attitude toward food! But attitude or not, those pangs are real as can be until you give your appetite to God.

What happened to me as a result of the happening that caused this book?
*I FEEL BETTER THAN I HAVE IN YEARS!
 *I HAVE MORE ENERGY THAN I'VE HAD IN YEARS!
  *THE FATIGUE I USED TO HAVE IS COMPLETELY
  GONE!
   *I DON'T WADDLE WITH JESUS, I CAN ACTUALLY
   WALK AND LEAP AND PRAISE GOD!
    *I LOOK 100% BETTER!

GOD'S ANSWER TO FAT . . . LOØSE IT!

*I CAN PASS BY THE WINDOW OF A STORE AND NOT BE ASHAMED OF THE WAY I LOOK.
*GONE IS THE GUILT OF BEING A FOODA-HOLIC!
*MY CLOTHES DON'T LOOK LIKE TENTS ANY MORE!
*I AM NO LONGER AN ENEMY OF THE CROSS OF CHRIST, BECAUSE NO LONGER IS MY GOD MY BELLY! THANK YOU, JESUS!!!
. . . . AND HE'LL DO THE SAME THING FOR YOU!

If you've read everything in this book so far, then I believe you REALLY mean business! And, if you really mean business, NOW is the time for us to get down to business and seriously pray. I know we've prayed before in this book, but some of the people fell by the wayside before they got this far, and so this is a very special prayer for all those who are going to stop kidding themselves. If you're one of those, please seriously pray with me right now (out loud) with all the earnestness that you possess.

"Dear Jesus, I am a foodaholic. I EAT TOO MUCH! I enjoy food too much. I eat to compensate for something lacking in my life, even though I don't know what it is. Dear Jesus, I HAVE NO WILL POWER. I know if I start on a diet right now I will stay on it for just a little while and then I'll go off of it, because I have no will power. I HAVE NO WILL POWER BECAUSE I AM A 'FOODAHOLIC' and I recognize this fact. Jesus, I'm going to give my food problem to you right now. I'm going to cast this care of mine on your shoulders, because you said that your yoke is easy and your burden is light. I'm going to trade you my appetite for your yoke which is easy. Jesus, now I'm going to do MY part. I'm going to seek ALL the wisdom and knowledge I can possibly find to let me know what I should and what I should not eat. I'm going to do all I can. Jesus, I ask you to give me that supernatural help I need. David cried out to you in his hour of need and you heard him. Right now I, wallowing in the middle of my fat and self-pity, ask you to give me the strength I need, the discipline I need, and the obedience I need to lose _____ pounds. I thank you right now, dear Jesus, for not letting me get tired, for not letting me think that the road is too long, for letting me believe that you can give me all the strength I need. Dear Jesus, I give you all the praise and all the glory because I pray and I believe in your beautiful and holy name."

That's the best ending you'll ever make, but it's really the beginning for you. If you really meant it, then you're going to learn all you can concerning calories! I want to remind you to check with your doctor and see what he says before you try any of the suggestions I have offered, because he will know what physical problems you may have. Also, I have made no attempt to define balance in food requirements — see your doctor and search for added knowledge to provide all the essentials your body needs. I will, too! Let's be real honest, however, and don't blame a BIG appetite on a physical problem. You might think it's a glandular problem, but it probably isn't! It's just a problem with your mouth. I know, because that was my problem! Hallelujah, but he set me free!

Let me suggest the purchase of two things, a postage scale to weigh food in your kitchen (A REAL MUST) and a good scale to weigh yourself on daily.

In Jesus name, I bind Satan, who has been controlling your appetite, right now in your life. I bind him, I cut off his power, and I loose the power of God in your life to take that fat off!

LOØSE IT . . . and let it go! And thank you for loving me when I was too overweight to be lovable!

Love,

Frances

Here's a chart you may find helpful in your food retraining program because it sets your GOAL FOR GOD
and each day you can see the goal getting smaller and
smaller. A real super thing is when you reach that point
where there's only 1 pound more to go, because when
that happens, you won't believe it went so fast, regardless of how hopeless it looks right now! Remember to
watch for the first 5 pounds, and then the next five!
Don't look at the overall loss that you need or you'll
get discouraged, look for the first five, then the second
five! It can be fun that way! Be sure and be honest on
the chart, because honesty will help YOU!

GOAL FOR GOD!   105

With God's help I want to lose _____ pounds.
Starting weight: _____

Date	Loss Today	Goal to Go for God	Total Calories	My Grade	Comments Why

Grade

A — Stayed with my desired Calorie investment
B — Cheated just a little bit
C — I weakened and ate that piece of _____
D — I blew it — Glutton Style

Food, approximate measure, and weight (in grams)			Water	Food energy	Protein	Carbohydrate

MILK, CHEESE, CREAM, IMITATION CREAM; RELATED PRODUCTS

		Grams	Percent	Calories	Grams	Grams
Milk:						
Fluid:						
Whole, 3.5% fat	1 cup	244	87	160	9	12
Nonfat (skim)	1 cup	245	90	90	9	12
Partly skimmed, 2% nonfat milk solids added.	1 cup	246	87	145	10	15
Canned, concentrated, undiluted:						
Evaporated, un- sweetened.	1 cup	252	74	345	18	24
Condensed, sweet- ened.	1 cup	306	27	980	25	166
Dry, nonfat instant:						
Low-density (1⅓ cups needed for re- constitution to 1 qt.).	1 cup	68	4	245	24	35
High-density (⅞ cup needed for recon- stitution to 1 qt.).	1 cup	104	4	375	37	54
Buttermilk:						
Fluid, cultured, made from skim milk.	1 cup	245	90	90	9	12
Dried, packaged	1 cup	120	3	465	41	60
Cheese:						
Natural:						
Blue or Roquefort type:						
Ounce	1 oz.	28	40	105	6	1
Cubic inch	1 cu. in.	17	40	65	4	Trace

Reproduced from Nutritive Value of Foods, Home and Garden Bulletin No. 72
UNITED STATES DEPARTMENT OF AGRICULTURE
U.S. GOVERNMENT PRINTING OFFICE
WASHINGTON, D.C. 20402

Food, approximate measure, and weight (in grams)			Water	Food energy	Pro-tein	Carbo-hy-drate
MILK, CHEESE, CREAM, IMITATION CREAM; RELATED PRODUCTS—Con.						
Cheese—Continued						
Natural—Continued		*Grams*	*Per-cent*	*Calo-ries*	*Grams*	*Grams*
Camembert, pack-aged in 4-oz. pkg. with 3 wedges per pkg.	1 wedge	38	52	115	7	1
Cheddar:						
Ounce	1 oz.	28	37	115	7	1
Cubic inch	1 cu. in.	17	37	70	4	Trace
Cottage, large or small curd:						
Creamed:						
Package of 12-oz., net wt.	1 pkg.	340	78	360	46	10
Cup, curd pressed down.	1 cup	245	78	260	33	7
Uncreamed:						
Package of 12-oz., net wt.	1 pkg.	340	79	290	58	9
Cup, curd pressed down.	1 cup	200	79	170	34	5
Cream:						
Package of 8-oz., net wt.	1 pkg.	227	51	850	18	5
Package of 3-oz., net wt.	1 pkg.	85	51	320	7	2
Cubic inch	1 cu. in.	16	51	60	1	Trace
Parmesan, grated:						
Cup, pressed down.	1 cup	140	17	655	60	5
Tablespoon	1 tbsp.	5	17	25	2	Trace
Ounce	1 oz.	28	17	130	12	1
Swiss:						
Ounce	1 oz.	28	39	105	8	1
Cubic inch	1 cu. in.	15	39	55	4	Trace

Pasteurized processed cheese:						
American:						
Ounce	1 oz.	28	40	105	7	1
Cubic inch	1 cu. in.	18	40	65	4	Trace
Swiss:						
Ounce	1 oz.	28	40	100	8	1
Cubic inch	1 cu. in.	.18	40	65	5	Trace
Pasteurized process cheese food, American:						
Tablespoon	1 tbsp.	14	43	45	3	1
Cubic inch	1 cu. in.	18	43	60	4	1
Pasteurized process cheese spread, American.	1 oz.	28	49	80	5	2
Cream:						
Half-and-half (cream and milk).	1 cup	242	80	325	8	11
	1 tbsp.	15	80	20	1	1
Light, coffee or table	1 cup	240	72	505	7	10
	1 tbsp.	15	72	30	1	1
Sour	1 cup	230	72	485	7	10
	1 tbsp.	12	72	25	Trace	1
Whipped topping (pressurized).	1 cup	60	62	155	2	6
	1 tbsp.	3	62	10	Trace	Trace
Whipping, unwhipped (volume about double when whipped):						
Light	1 cup	239	62	715	6	9
	1 tbsp.	15	62	45	Trace	1
Heavy	1 cup	238	57	840	5	7
	1 tbsp.	15	57	55	Trace	1
Imitation cream products (made with vegetable fat):						
Creamers:						
Powdered	1 cup	94	2	505	4	52
	1 tsp.	2	2	10	Trace	1
Liquid (frozen)	1 cup	245	77	345	3	25
	1 tbsp.	15	77	20	Trace	2
Sour dressing (imitation sour cream) made with nonfat dry milk.	1 cup	235	72	440	9	17
	1 tbsp.	12	72	20	Trace	1
Whipped topping:						
Pressurized	1 cup	70	61	190	1	9
	1 tbsp.	4	61	10	Trace	Trace

Food, approximate measure, and weight (in grams)			Water	Food energy	Pro- tein	Carbo- hy- drate
MILK, CHEESE, CREAM, IMITATION CREAM; RELATED PRODUCTS—Con.						
Whipped topping—Continued		*Grams*	*Per- cent*	*Calo- ries*	*Grams*	*Grams*
Frozen	1 cup	75	52	230	1	15
	1 tbsp.	4	52	10	Trace	1
Powdered, made with whole milk.	1 cup	75	58	175	3	15
	1 tbsp.	4	58	10	Trace	1
Milk beverages.						
Cocoa, homemade	1 cup	250	79	245	10	27
Chocolate-flavored drink made with skim milk and 2% added butterfat.	1 cup	250	83	190	8	27
Malted milk:						
Dry powder, approx. 3 heaping tea- spoons per ounce.	1 oz.	28	3	115	4	20
Beverage	1 cup	235	78	245	11	28
Milk desserts:						
Custard, baked	1 cup	265	77	305	14	29
Ice cream:						
Regular (approx. 10% fat).	½ gal.	1,064	63	2,055	48	221
	1 cup	133	63	255	6	28
	3 fl. oz. cup	50	63	95	2	10
Rich (approx. 16% fat).	½ gal.	1,188	63	2,635	31	214
	1 cup	148	63	330	4	27
Ice milk:						
Hardened	½ gal.	1,048	67	1,595	50	235
	1 cup	131	67	200	6	29
Soft-serve	1 cup	175	67	265	8	39

Yoghurt:					
Made from partially skimmed milk.	1 cup_____	245	89	125	8	13
Made from whole milk_	1 cup_____	245	88	150		12

EGGS

Eggs, large, 24 ounces per dozen:					
Raw or cooked in shell or with nothing added:					
Whole, without shell_	1 egg_____	50	74	80	6	Trace
White of egg_____	1 white_____	33	88	15	4	Trace
Yolk of egg_____	1 yolk_____	17	51	60	3	Trace
Scrambled with milk and fat.	1 egg_____	64	72	110	7	1

MEAT, POULTRY, FISH, SHELLFISH; RELATED PRODUCTS

Bacon, (20 slices per lb. raw), broiled or fried, crisp.	2 slices_____	15	8	90	5	1
Beef,[3] cooked:					
Cuts braised, simmered, or pot-roasted:					
Lean and fat_____	3 ounces_____	85	53	245	23	0
Lean only_____	2.5 ounces___	72	62	140	22	0
Hamburger (ground beef), broiled:					
Lean_____	3 ounces_____	85	60	185	23	0
Regular_____	3 ounces_____	85	54	245	21	0
Roast, oven-cooked, no liquid added:					
Relatively fat, such as rib:					
Lean and fat_____	3 ounces_____	85	40	375	17	0
Lean only_____	1.8 ounces___	51	57	125	14	0
Relatively lean, such as heel of round					
Lean and fat_____	3 ounces_____	85	62	165	25	0
Lean only_____	2.7 ounces__	78	65	125	24	0
Steak, broiled:					
Relatively, fat, such as sirloin:					
Lean and fat_____	3 ounces_____	85	44	330	20	0
Lean only_____	2.0 ounces___	56	59	115	18	0
Relatively, lean, such as round:					
Lean and fat_____	3 ounces_____	85	55	220	24	0
Lean only_ _____	2.4 ounces___	68	61	130	21	0
Beef, canned.					
Corned beef_____	3 ounces_____	85	59	185	22	0
Corned beef hash_____	3 ounces_____	85	67	155	7	9
Beef, dried or chipped____	2 ounces_____	57	48	115	19	0
Beef and vegetable stew__	1 cup_____	235	82	210	15	15

Food, approximate measure, and weight (in grams)			Water	Food energy	Pro-tein	Carbo-hy-drate

MEAT, POULTRY, FISH, SHELLFISH; RELATED PRODUCTS—Continued

		Grams	*Per-cent*	*Calo-ries*	*Grams*	*Grams*
Beef potpie, baked, 4¼-inch diam., weight before baking about 8 ounces.	1 pie_____	227	55	560	23	43
Chicken, cooked:						
Flesh only, broiled_____	3 ounces_____	85	71	115	20	0
Breast, fried, ½ breast:						
With bone_____	3.3 ounces___	94	58	155	25	1
Flesh and skin only__	2.7 ounces___	76	58	155	25	1
Drumstick, fried:						
With bone_____	2.1 ounces___	59	55	90	12	Trace
Flesh and skin only__	1.3 ounces___	38	55	90	12	Trace
Chicken, canned, boneless	3 ounces___	85	65	170	18	0
Chicken potpie, baked 4¼-inch diam., weight before baking about 8 ounces.	1 pie_____	227	57	535	23	42
Chili con carne, canned:						
With beans_____	1 cup_____	250	72	335	19	30
Without beans_____	1 cup_____	255	67	510	26	15
Heart, beef, lean, braised_	3 ounces_____	85	61	160	27	1
Lamb,[3] cooked:						
Chop, thick, with bone, broiled.	1 chop, 4.8 ounces.	137	47	400	25	0
Lean and fat_____	4.0 ounces___	112	47	400	25	0
Lean only_____	2.6 ounces___	74	62	140	21	0
Leg, roasted:						
Lean and fat_____	3 ounces_____	85	54	235	22	0
Lean only_____	2.5 ounces___	71	62	130	20	0
Shoulder, roasted:						
Lean and fat_____	3 ounces_____	85	50	285	18	0
Lean only_____	2.3 ounces___	64	61	130	17	0

Liver, beef, fried_____	2 ounces_____	57	57	130	15	3
Pork, cured, cooked:						
Ham, light cure, lean and fat, roasted.	3 ounces_____	85	54	245	18	0
Luncheon meat:						
Boiled ham, sliced___	2 ounces_____	57	59	135	11	0
Canned, spiced or unspiced.	2 ounces_____	57	55	165	8	1
Pork, fresh,[3] cooked:						
Chop, thick, with bone_	1 chop, 3.5 ounces.	98	42	260	16	0
Lean and fat_____	2.3 ounces___	66	42	260	16	0
Lean only_____	1.7 ounces___	48	53	130	15	0
Roast, oven-cooked, no liquid added:						
Lean and fat_____	3 ounces_____	85	46	310	21	0
Lean only_____	2.4 ounces___	68	55	175	20	0
Cuts, simmered:						
Lean and fat_____	3 ounces_____	85	46	320	20	0
Lean only_____	2.2 ounces___	63	60	135	18	0
Sausage:						
Bologna, slice, 3-in. diam. by ⅛ inch.	2 slices_____	26	56	80	3	Trace
Braunschweiger, slice 2-in. diam. by ¼ inch.	2 slices_____	20	53	65	3	Trace
Deviled ham, canned___	1 tbsp_____	13	51	45	2	0
Frankfurter, heated (8 per lb. purchased pkg.).	1 frank_____	56	57	170	7	1
Pork links, cooked (16 links per lb. raw).	2 links_____	26	35	125	5	Trace
Salami, dry type_____	1 oz_____	28	30	130	7	Trace
Salami, cooked_____	1 oz_____	28	51	90	5	Trace
Vienna, canned (7 sausages per 5-oz. can).	1 sausage____	16	63	40	2	Trace
Veal, medium fat, cooked, bone removed:						
Cutlet_____	3 oz_____	85	60	185	23	_____
Roast_____	3 oz_____	85	55	230	23	0
Fish and shellfish:						
Bluefish, baked with table fat.	3 oz_____	85	68	135	22	0
Clams:						
Raw, meat only_____	3 oz_____	85	82	65	11	2
Canned, solids and liquid.	3 oz_____	85	86	45	7	2
Crabmeat, canned_____	3 oz_____	85	77	85	15	1

Food, approximate measure, and weight (in grams)		Water	Food energy	Pro-tein	Carbo-hy-drate

MEAT, POULTRY, FISH, SHELLFISH; RELATED PRODUCTS—Continued

		Grams	*Per-cent*	*Calo-ries*	*Grams*	*Grams*
Fish and shellfish—Continued						
Fish sticks, breaded, cooked, frozen; stick 3¾ by 1 by ½ inch.	10 sticks or 8 oz. pkg.	227	66	400	38	15
Haddock, breaded, fried	3 oz.	85	66	140	17	5
Ocean perch, breaded, fried.	3 oz.	85	59	195	16	6
Oysters, raw, meat only (13–19 med. selects).	1 cup	240	85	160	20	8
Salmon, pink, canned	3 oz.	85	71	120	17	0
Sardines, Atlantic, canned in oil, drained solids.	3 oz.	85	62	175	20	0
Shad, baked with table fat and bacon.	3 oz.	85	64	170	20	0
Shrimp, canned, meat	3 oz.	85	70	100	21	1
Swordfish, broiled with butter or margarine.	3 oz.	85	65	150	24	0
Tuna, canned in oil, drained solids.	3 oz.	85	61	170	24	0

MATURE DRY BEANS AND PEAS, NUTS, PEANUTS; RELATED PRODUCTS

Almonds, shelled, whole kernels.	1 cup	142	5	850	26	28
Beans, dry: Common varieties as Great Northern, navy, and others: Cooked, drained: Great Northern	1 cup	180	69	210	14	38

Navy (pea)_____ 1 cup_____	190	69	225	15	40
Canned, solids and liquid:					
White with—					
Frankfurters 1 cup_____	255	71	365	19	32
(sliced).					
Pork and 1 cup_____	255	71	310	16	49
tomato sauce.					
Pork and sweet 1 cup_____	255	66	385	16	54
sauce.					
Red kidney_____ 1 cup_____	255	76	230	15	42
Lima, cooked, 1 cup_____	190	64	260	16	49
drained.					
Cashew nuts, roasted____ 1 cup_____	140	5	785	24	41
Coconut, fresh, meat only:					
Pieces, approx. 2 by 2 by 1 piece_____	45	51	155	2	4
½ inch.					
Shredded or grated, 1 cup_____	130	51	450	5	12
firmly packed.					
Cowpeas or blackeye 1 cup_____	248	80	190	13	34
peas, dry, cooked.					
Peanuts, roasted, 1 cup_____	144	2	840	37	27
salted, halves.					
Peanut butter_____ 1 tbsp._____	16	2	95	4	3
Peas, split, dry, cooked___ 1 cup_____	250	70	290	20	52
Pecans, halves_____ 1 cup_____	108	3	740	10	16
Walnuts, black or 1 cup_____	126	3	790	26	19
native, chopped.					
VEGETABLES AND VEGETABLE PRODUCTS					
Asparagus, green:					
Cooked, drained:					
Spears, ½-in. diam. 4 spears_____	60	94	10	1	2
at base.					
Pieces, 1½ to 2-in. 1 cup_____	145	94	30	3	5
lengths.					
Canned, solids and 1 cup_____	244	94	45	5	7
liquid.					
Beans:					
Lima, immature 1 cup_____	170	71	190	13	34
seeds, cooked, drained.					
Snap:					
Green:					
Cooked, drained___ 1 cup_____	125	92	30	2	7
Canned, solids 1 cup_____	239	94	45	2	10
and liquid.					

Food, approximate measure, and weight (in grams)			Water	Food energy	Pro-tein	Carbo-hy-drate

VEGETABLES AND VEGETABLE
PRODUCTS—Continued

		Grams	Per-cent	Calo-ries	Grams	Grams
Beans—Continued						
Snap—Continued						
Yellow or wax:						
Cooked, drained	1 cup	125	93	30	2	6
Canned, solids and liquid.	1 cup	239	94	45	2	10
Sprouted mung beans, cooked, drained.	1 cup	125	91	35	4	7
Beets:						
Cooked, drained, peeled:						
Whole beets, 2-in. diam.	2 beets	100	91	30	1	7
Diced or sliced	1 cup	170	91	55	2	12
Canned, solids and liquid.	1 cup	246	90	85	2	19
Beet greens, leaves and stems, cooked, drained.	1 cup	145	94	25	3	5
Blackeye peas. See Cowpeas.						
Broccoli, cooked, drained:						
Whole stalks, medium size.	1 stalk	180	91	45	6	8
Stalks cut into ½-in. pieces.	1 cup	155	91	40	5	7
Chopped, yield from 10-oz. frozen pkg.	1⅜ cups	250	92	65	7	12
Brussels sprouts, 7–8 sprouts (1¼ to 1½ in. diam.) per cup, cooked.	1 cup	155	88	55	7	10
Cabbage:						
Common varieties:						

Raw:					
Coarsely shredded or sliced.	1 cup_____	70	92	15	1	4
Finely shredded or chopped.	1 cup_____	90	92	20	1	5
Cooked_____	1 cup_____	145	94	30	2	6
Red, raw, coarsely shredded.	1 cup_____	70	90	20	1	5
Savoy, raw, coarsely shredded.	1 cup_____	70	92	15	2	3
Cabbage, celery or Chinese, raw, cut in 1-in. pieces.	1 cup_____	75	95	10	1	2
Cabbage, spoon (or pakchoy), cooked.	1 cup_____	170	95	25	2	4
Carrots:					
Raw:					
Whole, 5½ by 1 inch, (25 thin strips).	1 carrot_____	50	88	20	1	5
Grated_____	1 cup_____	110	88	45	1	11
Cooked, diced_____	1 cup_____	145	91	45	1	10
Canned, strained or chopped (baby food).	1 ounce_____	28	92	10	Trace	2
Cauliflower, cooked, flowerbuds.	1 cup_____	120	93	25	3	5
Celery, raw:					
Stalk, large outer, 8 by about 1½ inches, at root end.	1 stalk_____	40	94	5	Trace	2
Pieces, diced_____	1 cup_____	100	94	15	1	4
Collards, cooked_____	1 cup_____	190	91	55	5	9
Corn, sweet:					
Cooked, ear 5 by 1¾ inches.[5]	1 ear_____	140	74	70	3	16
Canned, solids and liquid.	1 cup_____	256	81	170	5	40
Cowpeas, cooked, immature seeds.	1 cup_____	160	72	175	13	29
Cucumbers, 10-ounce; 7½ by about 2 inches:					
Raw, pared_____	1 cucumber__	207	96	30	1	7
Raw, pared, center slice ⅛-inch thick.	6 slices_____	50	96	5	Trace	2
Dandelion greens, cooked_	1 cup_____	180	90	60	4	12

Food, approximate measure, and weight (in grams)		Water	Food energy	Pro- tein	Carbo- hy- drate

VEGETABLES AND VEGETABLE PRODUCTS—Continued

Food, approximate measure, and weight (in grams)		Water *Per- cent*	Food energy *Calo- ries*	Pro- tein *Grams*	Carbo- hydrate *Grams*
Endive, curly (including escarole).	2 ounces_____ *Grams* 57	93	10	1	2
Kale, leaves including stems, cooked.	1 cup_____ 110	91	30	4	4
Lettuce, raw:					
Butterhead, as Boston types; head, 4-inch diameter.	1 head_____ 220	95	30	3	6
Crisphead, as Iceberg; head, 4¾-inch diameter.	1 head_____ 454	96	60	4	13
Looseleaf, or bunching varieties, leaves.	2 large_____ 50	94	10	1	2
Mushrooms, canned, solids and liquid.	1 cup_____ 244	93	40	5	6
Mustard greens, cooked__	1 cup_____ 140	93	35	3	6
Okra, cooked, pod 3 by ⅝ inch.	8 pods_____ 85	91	25	2	5
Onions:					
Mature:					
Raw, onion 2½-inch diameter.	1 onion_____ 110	89	40	2	10
Cooked_____	1 cup_____ 210	92	60	3	14
Young green, small, without tops.	6 onions_____ 50	88	20	1	5
Parsley, raw, chopped____	1 tablespoon_ 4	85	Trace	Trace	Trace
Parsnips, cooked_____	1 cup_____ 155	82	100	?	23
Peas, green:					
Cooked_____	1 cup_____ 160	82	115	9	19
Canned, solids and liquid.	1 cup_____ 249	83	165	9	31

Food	Measure				
Canned, strained (baby food).	1 ounce_____	28	86	15	1	3
Peppers, hot, red, without seeds, dried (ground chili powder, added seasonings).	1 tablespoon_	15	8	50	2	8
Peppers, sweet:						
Raw, about 5 per pound:						
Green pod without stem and seeds.	1 pod_____	74	93	15	1	4
Cooked, boiled, drained	1 pod_____	73	95	15	1	3
Potatoes, medium (about 3 per pound raw):						
Baked, peeled after baking.	1 potato_____	99	75	90	3	21
Boiled:						
Peeled after boiling__	1 potato_____	136	80	105	3	23
Peeled before boiling_	1 potato_____	122	83	80	2	18
French-fried, piece 2 by ½ by ½ inch:						
Cooked in deep fat___	10 pieces____	57	45	155	2	20
Frozen, heated_____	10 pieces____	57	53	125	2	19
Mashed:						
Milk added_____	1 cup_____	195	83	125	4	25
Milk and butter added.	1 cup_____	195	80	185	4	24
Potato chips, medium, 2-inch diameter.	10 chips_____	20	2	115	1	10
Pumpkin, canned_____	1 cup_____	228	90	75	2	18
Radishes, raw, small, without tops.	4 radishes___	40	94	5	Trace	1
Sauerkraut, canned, solids and liquid.	1 cup_____	235	93	45	2	9
Spinach:						
Cooked_____	1 cup_____	180	92	40	5	6
Canned, drained solids_	1 cup_____	180	91	45	5	6
Squash:						
Cooked:						
Summer, diced_____	1 cup_____	210	96	30	2	7
Winter, baked, mashed.	1 cup_____	205	81	130	4	32
Sweetpotatoes:						
Cooked, medium, 5 by 2 inches, weight raw about 6 ounces:						
Baked, peeled after baking.	1 sweet-potato.	110	64	155	2	36
Boiled, peeled after boiling.	1 sweet-potato.	147	71	170	2	39

Food, approximate measure, and weight (in grams)		Water	Food energy	Pro- tein	Carbo- hy- drate
VEGETABLES AND VEGETABLE PRODUCTS—Continued					
Sweetpotatoes—Continued	*Grams*	*Per- cent*	*Calo- ries*	*Grams*	*Grams*
Candied, 3½ by 2¼ inches.	1 sweet- potato. 175	60	295	2	60
Canned, vacuum or solid pack.	1 cup_____ 218	72	235	4	54
Tomatoes:					
Raw, approx. 3-in. diam. 2⅛ in. high; wt., 7 oz.	1 tomato____ 200	94	40	2	9
Canned, solids and liquid.	1 cup_____ 241	94	50	2	10
Tomato catsup:					
Cup_____	1 cup_____ 273	69	290	6	69
Tablespoon_____	1 tbsp._____ 15	69	15	Trace	4
Tomato juice, canned:					
Cup_____	1 cup_____ 243	94	45	2	10
Glass (6 fl. oz.)_____	1 glass_____ 182	94	35	2	8
Turnips, cooked, diced___	1 cup_____ 155	94	35	1	8
Turnip greens, cooked____	1 cup_____ 145	94	30	3	5
FRUITS AND FRUIT PRODUCTS					
Apples, raw (about 3 per lb.).[5]	1 apple_____ 150	85	70	Trace	18
Apple juice, bottled or canned.	1 cup_____ 248	88	120	Trace	30
Applesauce, canned:					
Sweetened_____	1 cup_____ 255	76	230	1	61
Unsweetened or artifi- cially sweetened.	1 cup_____ 244	88	100	1	26

Apricots:					
Raw (about 12 per lb.) [5]	3 apricots____	114	85	55	1	14
Canned in heavy sirup__	1 cup_____	259	77	220	2	57
Dried, uncooked (40 halves per cup).	1 cup_____	150	25	390	8	100
Cooked, unsweetened, fruit and liquid.	1 cup_____	285	76	240	5	62
Apricot nectar, canned___	1 cup_____	251	85	140	1	37
Avocados, whole fruit, raw: [5]					
California (mid- and late-winter; diam. 3⅛ in.).	1 avocado___	284	74	370	5	13
Florida (late summer, fall; diam. 3⅝ in.).	1 avocado___	454	78	390	4	27
Bananas, raw, medium size.[5]	1 banana____	175	76	100	1	26
Banana flakes_____	1 cup_____	100	3	340	4	89
Blackberries, raw_____	1 cup_____	144	84	85	2	19
Blueberries, raw_____	1 cup_____	140	83	85	1	21
Cantaloups, raw; medium, 5-inch diameter about 1⅔ pounds.[5]	½ melon____	385	91	60	1	14
Cherries, canned, red, sour, pitted, water pack.	1 cup_____	244	88	105	2	26
Cranberry juice cocktail, canned.	1 cup_____	250	83	165	Trace	42
Cranberry sauce, sweetened, canned, strained.	1 cup_____	277	62	405	Trace	104
Dates, pitted, cut_____	1 cup_____	178	22	490	4	130
Figs, dried, large, 2 by 1 in.	1 fig_____	21	23	60	1	15
Fruit cocktail, canned, in heavy sirup.	1 cup_____	256	80	195	1	50

Food, approximate measure, and weight (in grams)		Water	Food energy	Pro-tein	Carbo-hy-drate

FRUITS AND FRUIT PRODUCTS—Con.

		Grams	Per-cent	Calo-ries	Grams	Grams
Grapefruit:						
Raw, medium, 3¾-in. diam.[5]						
White_____ ½ grape-fruit.		241	89	45	1	12
Pink or red _____ ½ grape-fruit.		241	89	50	1	13
Canned, sirup pack____ 1 cup_____		254	81	180	2	45
Grapefruit juice:						
Fresh_____ 1 cup_____		246	90	95	1	23
Canned, white:						
Unsweetened_____ 1 cup_____		247	89	100	1	24
Sweetened_____ 1 cup_____		250	86	130	1	32
Frozen, concentrate, unsweetened:						
Undiluted, can, 6 1 can_____ fluid ounces.		207	62	300	4	72
Diluted with 1 cup_____ 3 parts water, by volume.		247	89	100	1	24
Dehydrated crystals___ 4 oz_____		113	1	410	6	102
Prepared with water 1 cup_____ (1 pound yields about 1 gallon)		247	90	100	1	24
Grapes, raw: [5]						
American type (slip 1 cup_____ skin).		153	82	65	1	15
European type (ad- 1 cup_____ herent skin).		160	81	95	1	25
Grapejuice:						
Canned or bottled_____ 1 cup_____		253	83	165	1	42
Frozen concentrate, sweetened:						
Undiluted, can, 1 can_____ 6 fluid ounces.		216	53	395	1	100

Diluted with 3 parts water, by volume.	1 cup_____	250	86	135	1	33
Grapejuice drink, canned_	1 cup_____	250	86	135	Trace	35
Lemons, raw, 2⅛-in. diam., size 165.[5] Used for juice.	1 lemon_____	110	90	20	1	6
Lemon juice, raw_____	1 cup_____	244	91	60	1	20
Lemonade concentrate:						
Frozen, 6 fl. oz. per can_	1 can_____	219	48	430	Trace	112
Diluted with 4⅓ parts water, by volume.	1 cup_____	248	88	110	Trace	28
Lime juice:						
Fresh_____	1 cup_____	246	90	65	1	22
Canned, unsweetened__	1 cup_____	246	90	65	1	22
Limeade concentrate, frozen:						
Undiluted, can, 6 fluid ounces.	1 can_____	218	50	410	Trace	108
Diluted with 4⅓ parts water, by volume.	1 cup_____	247	90	100	Trace	27
Oranges, raw, 2⅝-in. diam., all commercial, varieties.[5]	1 orange_____	180	86	65	1	16
Orange juice, fresh, all varieties.	1 cup_____	248	88	110	2	26
Canned, unsweetened__	1 cup_____	249	87	120	2	28
Frozen concentrate:						
Undiluted, can, 6 fluid ounces.	1 can_____	213	55	360	5	87
Diluted with 3 parts water, by volume.	1 cup_____	249	87	120	2	29
Dehydrated crystals___	4 oz._____	113	1	430	6	100
Prepared with water (1 pound yields about 1 gallon).	1 cup_____	248	88	115	2	27
Orange-apricot juice drink	1 cup_____	249	87	125	1	32

FRUITS AND FRUIT PRODUCTS—Con.

Food, approximate measure, and weight (in grams)		Water	Food energy	Pro-tein	Carbo-hy-drate
	Grams	Per-cent	Calo-ries	Grams	Grams
Orange and grapefruit juice:					
Frozen concentrate:					
Undiluted, can, 6 fluid ounces.	1 can 210	59	330	4	78
Diluted with 3 parts water, by volume.	1 cup 248	88	110	1	26
Papayas, raw, ½-inch cubes.	1 cup 182	89	70	1	18
Peaches:					
Raw:					
Whole, medium, 2-inch diameter, about 4 per pound.[5]	1 peach 114	89	35	1	10
Sliced	1 cup 168	89	65	1	16
Canned, yellow-fleshed, solids and liquid:					
Sirup pack, heavy:					
Halves or slices	1 cup 257	79	200	1	52
Water pack	1 cup 245	91	75	1	20
Dried, uncooked	1 cup 160	25	420	5	109
Cooked, unsweet-ened, 10–12 halves and juice.	1 cup 270	77	220	3	58
Frozen:					
Carton, 12 ounces, not thawed.	1 carton 340	76	300	1	77
Pears:					
Raw, 3 by 2½-inch diameter.[5]	1 pear 182	83	100	1	25
Canned, solids and liquid:					
Sirup pack, heavy:					
Halves or slices	1 cup 255	80	195	1	50

Pineapple:					
Raw, diced_____	1 cup_____	140	85	75	1	19
Canned, heavy sirup pack, solids and liquid:					
Crushed_____	1 cup_____	260	80	195	1	50
Sliced, slices and	2 small or	122	80	90	Trace	24
juice.	1 large.					
Pineapple juice, canned___	1 cup_____	249	86	135	1	34
Plums, all except prunes:					
Raw, 2-inch diameter,	1 plum_____	60	87	25	Trace	7
about 2 ounces.[5]						
Canned, sirup pack (Italian prunes):					
Plums (with pits)	1 cup_____	256	77	205	1	53
and juice.[5]						
Prunes, dried, "softenized", medium:					
Uncooked [5]_____	4 prunes_____	32	28	70	1	18
Cooked, unsweetened,	1 cup_____	270	66	295	2	78
17–18 prunes and ⅓						
cup liquid.[5]						
Prune juice, canned or	1 cup_____	256	80	200	1	49
bottled.						
Raisins, seedless:					
Packaged, ½ oz. or	1 pkg._____	14	18	40	Trace	11
1½ tbsp. per pkg.						
Cup, pressed down____	1 cup_____	165	18	480	4	128
Raspberries, red:					
Raw_____	1 cup_____	123	84	70	1	17
Frozen, 10-ounce car-	1 carton_____	284	74	275	2	70
ton, not thawed.						
Rhubarb, cooked, sugar	1 cup_____	272	63	385	1	98
added.						
Strawberries:					
Raw, capped_____	1 cup_____	149	90	55	1	13
Frozen, 10-ounce car-	1 carton_____	284	71	310	1	79
ton, not thawed.						
Tangerines, raw, medium,	1 tangerine__	116	87	40	1	10
2⅜-in. diam., size 176.[5]						
Tangerine juice, canned,	1 cup_____	249	87	125	1	30
sweetened.						
Watermelon, raw, wedge,	1 wedge_____	925	93	115	2	27
4 by 8 inches (1/16 of 10						
by 16-inch melon, about						
2 pounds with rind).[5]						

Food, approximate measure, and weight (in grams)		Water	Food energy	Pro-tein	Carbo-hy-drate

GRAIN PRODUCTS

		Grams	Per-cent	Calo-ries	Grams	Grams
Bagel, 3-in. diam.:						
Egg	1 bagel	55	32	165	6	28
Water	1 bagel	55	29	165	6	30
Barley, pearled, light, uncooked.	1 cup	200	11	700	16	158
Biscuits, baking powder from home recipe with enriched flour, 2-in. diam.	1 biscuit	28	27	105	2	13
Biscuits, baking powder from mix, 2-in. diam.	1 biscuit	28	28	90	2	15
Bran flakes (40% bran), added thiamin and iron.	1 cup	35	3	105	4	28
Bran flakes with raisins, added thiamin and iron.	1 cup	50	7	145	4	40
Breads:						
Boston brown bread, slice 3 by ¾ in.	1 slice	48	45	100	3	22
Cracked-wheat bread:						
Loaf, 1 lb.	1 loaf	454	35	1,190	40	236
Slice, 18 slices per loaf.	1 slice	25	35	65	2	13
French or vienna bread:						
Enriched, 1 lb. loaf	1 loaf	454	31	1,315	41	251
Unenriched, 1 lb. loaf.	1 loaf	454	31	1,315	41	251
Italian bread:						
Enriched, 1 lb. loaf	1 loaf	454	32	1,250	41	256
Unenriched, 1 lb. loaf.	1 loaf	454	32	1,250	41	256
Raisin bread:						
Loaf, 1 lb.	1 loaf	454	35	1,190	30	243

Slice, 18 slices per loaf.	1 slice_____	25	35	65	2	13
Rye bread:						
American, light (⅓ rye, ⅔ wheat):						
Loaf, 1 lb._____	1 loaf_____	454	36	1,100	41	236
Slice, 18 slices per loaf.	1 slice_____	25	36	60	2	13
Pumpernickel, loaf, 1 lb.	1 loaf_____	454	34	1,115	41	241
White bread, enriched: [15]						
Soft-crumb type:						
Loaf, 1 lb._____	1 loaf_____	454	36	1,225	39	229
Slice, 18 slices per loaf.	1 slice_____	25	36	70	2	13
Slice, toasted___	1 slice_____	22	25	70	2	13
Slice, 22 slices per loaf.	1 slice_____	20	36	55	2	10
Slice, toasted____	1 slice_____	17	25	55	2	10
Loaf, 1½ lbs._____	1 loaf_____	680	36	1,835	59	343
Slice, 24 slices per loaf.	1 slice_____	28	36	75	2	14
Slice, toasted____	1 slice_____	24	25	75	2	14
Slice, 28 slices per loaf.	1 slice_____	24	36	65	2	12
Slice, toasted____	1 slice_____	21	25	65	2	12
Firm-crumb type:						
Loaf, 1 lb._____	1 loaf_____	454	35	1,245	41	228
Slice, 20 slices per loaf.	1 slice_____	23	35	65	2	12
Slice, toasted____	1 slice_____	20	24	65	2	12
Loaf, 2 lbs._____	1 loaf_ _____	907	35	2,495	82	455
Slice, 34 slices per loaf.	1 slice_____	27	35	75	2	14
Slice, toasted____	1 slice_____	23	35	75	2	14
Whole-wheat bread, soft-crumb type·						
Loaf, 1 lb._____	1 loaf_____	454	36	1,095	41	224
Slice, 16 slices per loaf.	1 slice_____	28	36	65	3	14
Slice, toasted_____	1 slice_____	24	24	65	3	14

Food, approximate measure, and weight (in grams)			Water	Food energy	Protein	Carbohydrate
GRAIN PRODUCTS—Continued						
Bread—Continued		*Grams*	*Percent*	*Calories*	*Grams*	*Grams*
Whole-wheat bread, firm-crumb type:						
Loaf, 1 lb.	1 loaf	454	36	1,100	48	216
Slice, 18 slices per loaf.	1 slice	25	36	60	3	12
Slice, toasted	1 slice	21	24	60	3	12
Breadcrumbs, dry, grated.	1 cup	100	6	390	13	73
Buckwheat flour, light, sifted.	1 cup	98	12	340	6	78
Bulgur, canned, seasoned.	1 cup	135	56	245	8	44
Cakes made from cake mixes:						
Angelfood:						
Whole cake	1 cake	635	34	1,645	36	377
Piece, ¹⁄₁₂ of 10-in. diam. cake.	1 piece	53	34	135	3	32
Cupcakes, small, 2½ in. diam.:						
Without icing	1 cupcake	25	26	90	1	14
With chocolate icing.	1 cupcake	36	22	130	2	21
Devil's food, 2-layer, with chocolate icing:						
Whole cake	1 cake	1,107	24	3,755	49	645
Piece, ¹⁄₁₆ of 9-in. diam. cake.	1 piece	69	24	235	3	40
Cupcake, small, 2½ in. diam.	1 cupcake	35	24	120	2	20
Gingerbread:						
Whole cake	1 cake	570	37	1,575	18	291
Piece, ⅑ of 8-in. square cake.	1 piece	63	37	175	2	32
White, 2-layer, with chocolate icing:						
Whole cake	1 cake	1,140	21	4,000	45	716

Food	Measure					
Piece, 1/16 of 9-in. diam. cake.	1 piece	71	21	250	3	45
Cakes made from home recipes: [16]						
Boston cream pie; piece 1/12 of 8-in. diam.	1 piece	69	35	210	4	34
Fruitcake, dark, made with enriched flour:						
Loaf, 1-lb.	1 loaf	454	18	1,720	22	271
Slice, 1/30 of 8-in. loaf.	1 slice	15	18	55	1	9
Plain sheet cake:						
Without icing:						
Whole cake	1 cake	777	25	2,830	35	434
Piece, 1/9 of 9-in. square cake.	1 piece	86	25	315	4	48
With boiled white icing, piece, 1/9 of 9-in. square cake.	1 piece	114	23	400	4	71
Pound:						
Loaf, 8½ by 3½ by 3in.	1 loaf	514	17	2,430	29	242
Slice, ½-in. thick	1 slice	30	17	140	2	14
Sponge:						
Whole cake	1 cake	790	32	2,345	60	427
Piece, 1/12 of 10-in. diam. cake.	1 piece	66	32	195	5	36
Yellow, 2-layer, without icing:						
Whole cake	1 cake	870	24	3,160	39	506
Piece, 1/16 of 9-in. diam. cake.	1 piece	54	24	200	2	32
Yellow, 2-layer, with chocolate icing:						
Whole cake	1 cake	1,203	21	4,390	51	727
Piece, 1/16 of 9-in. diam. cake.	1 piece	75	21	275	3	45
Cake icings. See Sugars, Sweets.						
Cookies:						
Brownies with nuts:						
Made from home recipe with enriched flour.	1 brownie	20	10	95	1	10
Made from mix	1 brownie	20	11	85	1	13

Food, approximate measure, and weight (in grams)			Water	Food energy	Pro- tein	Carbo- hy- drate

GRAIN PRODUCTS—Continued

		Grams	*Per- cent*	*Calo- ries*	*Grams*	*Grams*
Cookies—Continued						
Chocolate chip:						
Made from home recipe with en- riched flour.	1 cookie_ _ _	10	3	50	1	6
Commercial_____	1 cookie_____	10	3	50	1	7
Fig bars, commercial___	1 cookie__ __	14	14	50	1	11
Sandwich, chocolate or vanilla, commercial.	1 cookie_ ___	10	2	50	1	7
Corn flakes, added nutrients:						
Plain_____	1 cup_____	25	4	100	2	21
Sugar-covered_____	1 cup_____	40	2	155	2	36
Corn (hominy) grits, degermed, cooked:						
Enriched_____ _____	1 cup_____	245	87	125	3	27
Unenriched_____	1 cup_____	245	87	125	3	27
Cornmeal:						
Whole-ground, unbolted, dry.	1 cup__ ____	122	12	435	11	90
Bolted (nearly whole- grain) dry.	1 cup__ ___	122	12	440	11	91
Degermed, enriched:						
Dry form_____	1 cup_____	138	12	500	11	108
Cooked_____	1 cup_____	240	88	120	3	26
Degermed, unenriched:						
Dry form_____	1 cup_____	138	12	500	11	108
Cooked_____	1 cup_____	240	88	120	3	26
Corn muffins, made with enriched de- germed cornmeal and enriched flour; muffin 2⅜-in. diam.	1 muffin ____	40	33	125	3	19

Corn muffins, made with mix, egg, and milk; muffin 2⅜-in. diam.	1 muffin	40	30	130	3	20
Corn, puffed, presweetened, added nutrients.	1 cup	30	2	115	1	27
Corn, shredded, added nutrients.	1 cup	25	3	100	2	22
Crackers:						
Graham, 2½-in. square.	4 crackers	28	6	110	2	21
Saltines	4 crackers	11	4	50	1	8
Danish pastry, plain (without fruit or nuts):						
Packaged ring, 12 ounces.	1 ring	340	22	1,435	25	155
Round piece, approx. 4¼-in. diam. by 1 in.	1 pastry	65	22	275	5	30
Ounce	1 oz.	28	22	120	2	13
Doughnuts, cake type	1 doughnut	32	24	125	1	16
Farina, quick-cooking, enriched, cooked.	1 cup	245	89	105	3	22
Macaroni, cooked:						
Enriched:						
Cooked, firm stage (undergoes additional cooking in a food mixture).	1 cup	130	64	190	6	39
Cooked until tender	1 cup	140	72	155	5	32
Unenriched:						
Cooked, firm stage (undergoes additional cooking in a food mixture).	1 cup	130	64	190	6	39
Cooked until tender	1 cup	140	72	155	5	32
Macaroni (enriched) and cheese, baked.	1 cup	200	58	430	17	40
Canned	1 cup	240	80	230	9	26
Muffins, with enriched white flour; muffin, 3-inch diam.	1 muffin	40	38	120	3	17
Noodles (egg noodles), cooked:						
Enriched	1 cup	160	70	200	7	37
Unenriched	1 cup	160	70	200	7	37

Food, approximate measure, and weight (in grams)		Water	Food energy	Protein	Carbohydrate
GRAIN PRODUCTS—Continued					
	Grams	Percent	Calories	Grams	Grams
Oats (with or without corn) puffed, added nutrients.	1 cup_____ 25	3	100	3	19
Oatmeal or rolled oats, cooked.	1 cup_____ 240	87	130	5	23
Pancakes, 4-inch diam.:					
Wheat, enriched flour (home recipe).	1 cake_____ 27	50	60	2	9
Buckwheat (made from mix with egg and milk).	1 cake_____ 27	58	55	2	6
Plain or buttermilk (made from mix with egg and milk).	1 cake_____ 27	51	60	2	9
Pie (piecrust made with unenriched flour):					
Sector, 4-in., ⅐ of 9-in. diam. pie:					
Apple (2-crust)_____	1 sector_____ 135	48	350	3	51
Butterscotch (1-crust)__	1 sector_____ 130	45	350	6	50
Cherry (2-crust)_____	1 sector_____ 135	47	350	4	52
Custard (1-crust)_____	1 sector_____ 130	58	285	8	30
Lemon meringue (1-crust).	1 sector_____ 120	47	305	4	45
Mince (2-crust)_____	1 sector_____ 135	43	365	3	56
Pecan (1-crust)_____	1 sector_____ 118	20	490	6	60
Pineapple chiffon (1-crust).	1 sector_____ 93	41	265	6	36
Pumpkin (1-crust)_____	1 sector_____ 130	59	275	5	32
Piecrust, baked shell for pie made with:					
Enriched flour_____	1 shell_____ 180	15	900	11	79
Unenriched flour_____	1 shell_____ 180	15	900	11	79

Piecrust mix including stick form:					
Package, 10-oz., for double crust.	1 pkg.	284	9	1,480	20	141
Pizza (cheese) 5½-in. sector; ⅛ of 14-in. diam. pie.	1 sector	75	45	185	7	27
Popcorn, popped:					
Plain, large kernel	1 cup	6	4	25	1	5
With oil and salt	1 cup	9	3	40	1	5
Sugar coated	1 cup	35	4	135	2	30
Pretzels:					
Dutch, twisted	1 pretzel	16	5	60	2	12
Thin, twisted	1 pretzel	6	5	25	1	5
Stick, small, 2¼ inches.	10 sticks	3	5	10	Trace	2
Stick, regular, 3⅛ inches.	5 sticks	3	5	10	Trace	2
Rice, white:					
Enriched:					
Raw	1 cup	185	12	670	12	149
Cooked	1 cup	205	73	225	4	50
Instant, ready-to-serve.	1 cup	165	73	180	4	40
Unenriched, cooked	1 cup	205	73	225	4	50
Parboiled, cooked	1 cup	175	73	185	4	41
Rice, puffed, added nutrients.	1 cup	15	4	60	1	13
Rolls, enriched:					
Cloverleaf or pan:					
Home recipe	1 roll	35	26	120	3	20
Commercial	1 roll	28	31	85	2	15
Frankfurter or hamburger.	1 roll	40	31	120	3	21
Hard, round or rectangular.	1 roll	50	25	155	5	30
Rye wafers, whole-grain, 1⅞ by 3½ inches.	2 wafers	13	6	45	2	10
Spaghetti, cooked, tender stage, enriched.	1 cup	140	72	155	5	32

Food, approximate measure, and weight (in grams)		Water	Food energy	Pro- tein	Carbo- hy- drate

GRAIN PRODUCTS—Continued

	Grams	Per- cent	Calo- ries	Grams	Grams
Spaghetti with meat balls, and tomato sauce:					
Home recipe_____ 1 cup_____	248	70	330	19	39
Canned_____ 1 cup_____	250	78	260	12	28
Spaghetti in tomato sauce with cheese:					
Home recipe_____ 1 cup_____	250	77	260	9	37
Canned_____ 1 cup_____	250	80	190	6	38
Waffles, with enriched 1 waffle_____ flour, 7-in. diam.	75	41	210	7	28
Waffles, made from mix, 1 waffle_____ enriched, egg and milk added, 7-in. diam.	75	42	205	7	27
Wheat, puffed, added 1 cup_____ nutrients.	15	3	55	2	12
Wheat, shredded, plain___ 1 biscuit_____	25	7	90	2	20
Wheat flakes, added 1 cup_____ nutrients.	30	4	105	3	24
Wheat flours:					
Whole-wheat, from 1 cup_____ hard wheats, stirred.	120	12	400	16	85
All-purpose or family flour, enriched:					
Sifted_____ 1 cup_____	115	12	420	12	88
Unsifted_____ 1 cup_____	125	12	455	13	95
Self-rising, enriched____ 1 cup_____	125	12	440	12	93
Cake or pastry flour, 1 cup_____ sifted.	96	12	350	7	76

FATS, OILS

Butter:					
Regular, 4 sticks per pound:					
Stick_____ ½ cup_____	113	16	810	1	1

Tablespoon (approx. ⅛ stick).	1 tbsp.	14	16	100	Trace	Trace
Pat (1-in. sq. ⅓-in. high; 90 per lb.).	1 pat	5	16	35	Trace	Trace
Whipped, 6 sticks or 2, 8-oz. containers per pound:						
Stick	½ cup	76	16	540	1	Trace
Tablespoon (approx. ⅛ stick).	1 tbsp.	9	16	65	Trace	Trace
Pat (1¼-in. sq. ⅓-in. high; 120 per lb.).	1 pat	4	16	25	Trace	Trace
Fats, cooking:						
Lard	1 cup	205	0	1,850	0	0
	1 tbsp.	13	0	115	0	0
Vegetable fats	1 cup	200	0	1,770	0	0
	1 tbsp.	13	0	110	0	0
Margarine:						
Regular, 4 sticks per pound:						
Stick	½ cup	113	16	815	1	1
Tablespoon (approx. ⅛ stick).	1 tbsp.	14	16	100	Trace	Trace
Pat (1-in. sq. ⅓-in. high; 90 per lb.).	1 pat	5	16	35	Trace	Trace
Whipped, 6 sticks per pound:						
Stick	½ cup	76	16	545	1	Trace
Soft, 2 8-oz. tubs per pound:						
Tub	1 tub	227	16	1,635	1	1
Tablespoon	1 tbsp.	14	16	100	Trace	Trace
Oils, salad or cooking:						
Corn	1 cup	220	0	1,945	0	0
	1 tbsp.	14	0	125	0	0
Cottonseed	1 cup	220	0	1,945	0	0
	1 tbsp.	14	0	125	0	0
Olive	1 cup	220	0	1,945	0	0
	1 tbsp.	14	0	125	0	0
Peanut	1 cup	220	0	1,945	0	0
	1 tbsp.	14	0	125	0	0
Safflower	1 cup	220	0	1,945	0	0
	1 tbsp.	14	0	125	0	0
Soybean	1 cup	220	0	1,945	0	0
	1 tbsp.	14	0	125	0	0

Food, approximate measure, and weight (in grams)		Water	Food energy	Pro-tein	Carbo-hy-drate
FATS, OILS—Continued					
	Grams	*Per-cent*	*Calo-ries*	*Grams*	*Grams*
Salad dressings:					
Blue cheese_____ 1 tbsp._____	15	32	75	1	1
Commercial, mayonnaise type:					
Regular_____ 1 tbsp._____	15	41	65	Trace	2
Special dietary, low- 1 tbsp._____ calorie.	16	81	20	Trace	1
French:					
Regular_____ 1 tbsp._____	16	39	65	Trace	3
Special dietary, low- 1 tbsp._____ fat with artificial sweeteners.	15	95	Trace	Trace	Trace
Home cooked, boiled_____ 1 tbsp._____	16	68	25	1	2
Mayonnaise_____ 1 tbsp._____	14	15	100	Trace	Trace
Thousand island_____ 1 tbsp._____	16	32	80	Trace	3
SUGARS, SWEETS					
Cake icings:					
Chocolate made with 1 cup_____ milk and table fat.	275	14	1,035	9	185
Coconut (with boiled 1 cup_____ icing).	166	15	605	3	124
Creamy fudge from 1 cup_____ mix with water only.	245	15	830	7	183
White, boiled_____ 1 cup_____	94	18	300	1	76
Candy:					
Caramels, plain or 1 oz._____ chocolate.	28	8	115	1	22
Chocolate, milk, plain__ 1 oz._____	28	1	145	2	16
Chocolate-coated 1 oz._____ peanuts.	28	1	160	5	11

Fondant; mints, un-coated; candy corn.	1 oz.	28	8	105	Trace	25
Fudge, plain	1 oz.	28	8	115	1	21
Gum drops	1 oz.	28	12	100	Trace	25
Hard	1 oz.	28	1	110	0	28
Marshmallows	1 oz.	28	17	90	1	23
Chocolate-flavored sirup or topping:						
Thin type	1 fl. oz.	38	32	90	1	24
Fudge type	1 fl. oz.	38	25	125	2	20
Chocolate-flavored beverage powder (approx. 4 heaping teaspoons per oz.):						
With nonfat dry milk	1 oz.	28	2	100	5	20
Without nonfat dry milk.	1 oz.	28	1	100	1	25
Honey, strained or extracted.	1 tbsp.	21	17	65	Trace	17
Jams and preserves	1 tbsp.	20	29	55	Trace	14
Jellies	1 tbsp.	18	29	50	Trace	13
Molasses, cane:						
Light (first extraction)	1 tbsp.	20	24	50	------	13
Blackstrap (third extraction).	1 tbsp.	20	24	45	------	11
Sirups:						
Sorghum	1 tbsp.	21	23	55	------	14
Table blends, chiefly corn, light and dark.	1 tbsp.	21	24	60	0	15
Sugars:						
Brown, firm packed	1 cup	220	2	820	0	212
White:						
Granulated	1 cup	200	Trace	770	0	199
	1 tbsp.	11	Trace	40	0	11
Powdered, stirred before measuring.	1 cup	120	Trace	460	0	119

MISCELLANEOUS ITEMS

Barbecue sauce	1 cup	250	81	230	4	20
Beverages, alcoholic:						
Beer	12 fl. oz.	360	92	150	1	14
Gin, rum, vodka, whiskey:						
80-proof	1½ fl. oz. jigger.	42	67	100	------	Trace
86-proof	1½ fl. oz. jigger.	42	64	105	------	Trace
90-proof	1½ fl. oz. jigger.	42	62	110	------	Trace

Food, approximate measure, and weight (in grams)	Water	Food energy	Protein	Carbohydrate

MISCELLANEOUS ITEMS—Continued

	Grams	Per cent	Calories	Grams	Grams
Beverages, alcoholic—Continued					
Gin, rum, vodka, whiskey—Con.					
94-proof ___ 1½ fl. oz. jigger.	42	60	115	------	Trace
100-proof ___ 1½ fl. oz. jigger.	42	58	125	------	Trace
Wines:					
Dessert ___ 3½ fl. oz. glass.	103		140	Trace	8
Table ___ 3½ fl. oz. glass.	102	86	85	Trace	4
Beverages, carbonated, sweetened, nonalcoholic:					
Carbonated water ___ 12 fl. oz.	366	92	115	0	29
Cola type ___ 12 fl. oz.	369	90	145	0	37
Fruit-flavored sodas and Tom Collins mixes. ___ 12 fl. oz.	372	88	170	0	45
Ginger ale ___ 12 fl. oz.	366	92	115	0	29
Root beer ___ 12 fl. oz.	370	90	150	0	39
Bouillon cubes, approx. ½ in. ___ 1 cube	4	4	5	1	Trace
Chocolate:					
Bitter or baking ___ 1 oz.	28	2	145	3	8
Semi-sweet, small pieces. ___ 1 cup	170	1	860	7	97
Gelatin:					
Plain, dry powder in envelope. ___ 1 envelope	7	13	25	6	0
Dessert powder, 3-oz. package. ___ 1 pkg.	85	2	315	8	75
Gelatin dessert, prepared with water. ___ 1 cup	240	84	140	4	34

NON CHRISTIAN

Olives, pickled:					
Green_____	4 medium or 3 extra large or 2 giant.	16	78	15	Trace	Trace
Ripe: Mission_____	3 small or 2 large.	10	73	15	Trace	Trace
Pickles, cucumber:					
Dill, medium, whole, 3¾ in. long, 1¼ in. diam.	1 pickle_____	65	93	10	1	1
Fresh, sliced, 1½ in. diam., ¼ in. thick.	2 slices_____	15	79	10	Trace	3
Sweet, gherkin, small, whole, approx. 2½ in. long, ¾ in. diam.	1 pickle_____	15	61	20	Trace	6
Relish, finely chopped, sweet.	1 tbsp._____	15	63	20	Trace	5
Popcorn. See Grain Products.					
Popsicle, 3 fl. oz. size____	1 popsicle____	95	80	70	0	18
Pudding, home recipe with starch base:					
Chocolate_____	1 cup_____	260	66	385	8	67
Vanilla (blanc mange)__	1 cup_____	255	76	285	9	41
Pudding mix, dry form, 4-oz. package.	1 pkg___ ____	113	2	410	3	103
Sherbet_____	1 cup_____	193	67	260	2	59
Soups:					
Canned, condensed, ready-to-serve:					
Prepared with an equal volume of milk:					
Cream of chicken__	1 cup_____	245	85	180	7	15
Cream of mush-room.	1 cup_ _____	245	83	215	7	16
Tomato_____	1 cup_____	250	84	175	7	23
Prepared with an equal volume of water:					
Bean with pork___	1 cup_____	250	84	170	8	22
Beef broth, bouil-lon consomme.	1 cup_____	240	96	30	5	3
Beef noodle_____	1 cup_____	240	93	70	4	7
Clam chowder, Manhattan type (with tomatoes, without milk).	1 cup_____	245	92	80	2	12
Cream of chicken__	1 cup_____	240	92	95	3	8
Cream of mush-room.	1 cup_____	240	90	135	2	10
Minestrone_____	1 cup_____	245	90	105	5	14

Food, approximate measure, and weight (in grams)	Water	Food energy	Pro-tein	Carbo-hy-drate
MISCELLANEOUS ITEMS—Continued				
Soups—Continued				
Canned, condensed, ready-to-serve—Con.				
Prepared with an equal volume of	*Per-cent*	*Calo-ries*	*Grams*	*Grams*
water—Con. *Grams*				
Split pea_____ 1 cup_____ 245	85	145	9	21
Tomato_____ 1 cup_____ 245	90	90	2	16
Vegetable beef____ 1 cup_____ 245	92	80	5	10
Vegetarian_____ 1 cup_____ 245	92	80	2	13
Dehydrated, dry form:				
Chicken noodle 1 pkg._____ 57	6	220	8	33
(2-oz. package).				
Onion mix (1½-oz. 1 pkg._____ 43	3	150	6	23
package).				
Tomato vegetable 1 pkg._____ 71	4	245	6	45
with noodles (2½-oz. pkg.).				
Frozen, condensed:				
Clam chowder, New England type (with milk, without tomatoes):				
Prepared with 1 cup_____ 245	83	210	9	16
equal volume of milk.				
Prepared with 1 cup_____ 240	89	130	4	11
equal volume of water.				
Cream of potato:				
Prepared with 1 cup_____ 245	83	185	8	18
equal volume of milk.				
Prepared with 1 cup_____ 240	90	105	3	12
equal volume of water.				

Cream of shrimp:					
Prepared with equal volume of milk.	1 cup	245	82	245	9	15
Prepared with equal volume of water.	1 cup	240	88	160	5	8
Oyster stew:					
Prepared with equal volume of milk.	1 cup	240	83	200	10	14
Prepared with equal volume of water.	1 cup	240	90	120	6	8
Tapioca, dry, quick-cooking.	1 cup	152	13	535	1	131
Tapioca desserts:					
Apple	1 cup	250	70	295	1	74
Cream pudding	1 cup	165	72	220	8	28
Tartar sauce	1 tbsp.	14	34	75	Trace	1
Vinegar	1 tbsp.	15	94	Trace	Trace	1
White sauce, medium	1 cup	250	73	405	10	22
Yeast:					
Baker's, dry, active	1 pkg.	7	5	20	3	3
Brewer's, dry	1 tbsp.	8	5	25	3	3
Yoghurt. See Milk, Cheese, Cream, Imitation Cream.					

Reproduced from Nutritive Value of Foods,
Home and Garden Bulletin No. 72
UNITED STATES DEPARTMENT OF AGRICULTURE
U.S. GOVERNMENT PRINTING OFFICE
WASHINGTON, D.C. 20402

CHAPTER XIII

SKINNY MINNIE RECIPES

Get your imagination ready to work, because if you really are serious about a food retraining program, God will drop into your mind some interesting things to eat and unique ways to prepare them. I'm giving you just a starter in a few different areas, but I think if you'll experiment you'll enjoy your own creations! We've really had fun discovering the new dishes we can eat with very few calories which are delightful! Make it a challenge and not a drag!

MUSHROOM CHICKEN (Serves 4)

	Calories per person
4 Chicken Breasts (avg. 5 ounces ea)	175
1 cup fresh mushrooms	10
1 tbsp. soy sauce	1
1 pat butter	9
dehydrated parsley	—
paprika	—
	Total calories 195

Lay chicken breasts in bottom of casserole dish, add soy sauce, butter and dehydrated parsley. Sprinkle salt, pepper and paprika on top of chicken. Bake at 450 degrees for 20 minutes. Add mushrooms for the last 5 minutes.

FISH DELIGHT

3 ounces whitefish (poached) 150
slice lemon
mushrooms (½ cup) 20
tabasco sauce
dill weed
Reducer's French Dressing, 1 Tbsp........................   2

Poach the fish for 20 minutes in boiling water with slice of lemon added, place in baking dish and add 1/2 cup mushrooms, sprinkling of dill weed. Mix two or three drops tabasco sauce with French dressing and 1 tbsp. water, heat and pour over fish. To remove "fishy" taste, soak fish in salt water and ice cubes for 20 to 30 minutes before preparing.

PAKISTAN VEGETABLE CURRY

2 cups chopped onion
2 cups diced potato
2 cups cauliflower
1 cup green pepper cut in strips
1 cup chopped celery
1 heaping teaspoon finely chopped garlic
2 tablespoons imported curry powder
1 tablespoon chili powder
salt to taste

Brown curry powder in dry skillet until light brown; remove curry from skillet; spray skillet with no stick vegetable spray, saute onions until golden; add garlic and saute another minute or two. Place curry, onions and garlic in a deep pot, add 1 quart of water and bring to a boil; add potatoes and cook over medium heat until almost done, then add celery, peppers and finally, cauliflower. The object is to serve the curry when potatoes and celery are done but cauliflower and peppers are still firm. To thicken gravy, withhold some water, or add instant potato flakes.

Serves 6 people (105 calories per serving)

This delightful recipe was concocted by Jim Wheeless of Hunter Ministries.

FARMER'S CHEESE

One of the best "no fat" foods I know of is "pot" cheese or "Farmer's Cheese" because of the variety of ways you can fix it. It may take a little "getting used to" because of the different flavor, but the lack of calories makes it worth while!

1 8 oz. package Farmer's Cheese
1 hard boiled egg, grated
1 teas. Soy Sauce
½ teas. chopped chives
Season Salt to taste
¼ cup water

Since Farmer's Cheese is very dry, add about ¼ cup water before you add the rest of the ingredients. Then mix together and let sit overnight so the flavor comes through. Excellent when eaten with Seasoned Rye Krisp or Sesame Seed Breadsticks. May also add 2 T Reducer's Mayonnaise.

1 8 oz. package Farmer's Cheese
1 teas. regular mustard
1 teas. horseradish
¼ teas. celery seed
¼ cup water
Season salt to taste

1 8 oz. package Farmer's Cheese
2 Tbls. Taco Sauce
Season Salt to Taste

1 8 oz. package Farmer's Cheese
¼ cup water
2 teas. artificial sweetner
Cinnamon to taste

Put on top of rye crisp (heaped up) and then put under broiler for few minutes. Good for those who have a sweet taste. For variety, add a couple of thin slices of apple before broiling. Takes a little getting used to in the beginning, but keeps the hunger pangs down.

SHRIMP COCKTAIL

1 can medium deveined shrimp
1 Tbls. Soy Sauce
½ lemon, squeezed

Drain shrimp, wash so that all "fishy" taste is removed. Put in container with ice for 30 minutes. Drain, and serve with Soy Sauce & lemon.

LEMON PEPPER CABBAGE

1 head cabbage (medium size). Cut into small chunks
Put 4 Tablespoons of any kind Reducer's Dressing into skillet
    (I like either French or Remoulade)
Add 4 Tablespoons of water

Bring liquid to a fast boil, add cabbage, and then sprinkle a supply of Lemon Pepper on top. Not too much, but enough so you can see it, and it will give a spicy taste. Stir fry, until cabbage is slightly transparent (approximately 4 minutes). Crisp enough to be delicious, but done enough to taste good enough for a King! (Your husband)

SOY-STIR CELERY AND ONIONS

Clean 1 stalk celery and cut at angle into pieces about ½" wide
Cut 5 big onions into small chunks
Season Salt to taste

Put 4 Tablespoons of water into skillet, add 4 Tablespoons of Soy Sauce. Stir fry until celery has faint transparent look (approximately 4 minutes). Remove from stove and add extra soy sauce if needed. Let sit approximately 5 minutes before serving.

SPICY FISH

USE 1 pound fish fillets (any kind). Place in bottom of baking dish.
Add 1 small can spicy tomato juice
Add 4 thin slices onion and lay on top. Put one lemon circle on top
Bake for 25 minutes at 350 degrees

HAMBURGER

If you have a craving for beef, try 1 lb. hamburger seasoned with salt, pepper, and a small amount of onions if you like. (Mushrooms are a good substitute, too). Stir continually until hamburger crumbles and is completely done. DRAIN ALL THE FAT OFF. Add 1 Tablespoon Soy Sauce to replace flavor. Serve immediately!

It might surprise you to know that you can have a very unique breakfast, which will completely eliminate the luncheon meal during the day; and yet you'll have a very small amount of calories. This is my breakfast most of the time:

One slice of bacon	45 calories
Two poached eggs (or boiled)	160 calories
One 3-oz. baked potato	51 calories
	256 calories

Even on the most restricted of diets, 256 calories for one of two meals for the day isn't bad at all. Try this tomorrow morning and see what happens to your appetite. And by the way, looking at my daily breakfast, I think it's interesting that it all started with potatoes, and now it's ending with potatoes!

In trying to find the right balance for me to eat without continuing to lose weight, and without gaining weight back again, I eat what I need of all different kinds of foods, but I am very conscious of the fact it's the little things that create the BIG problems!

*LEAVE OFF THE SALAD DRESSING
*CUT OUT THE BREAD, then you won't have anything to put the butter and jelly on
*LEAVE OUT THE OILS AND BUTTER
*SKIP THAT SUPER SWEET DESSERT!
and remember to give the glory to God!